The ULTIMATE MUFFIN Book

OTHER BOOKS BY BRUCE WEINSTEIN

The Ultimate Candy Book

The Ultimate Ice Cream Book

The Ultimate Party Drink Book

OTHER BOOKS BY BRUCE WEINSTEIN AND MARK SCARBROUGH

Cooking for Two

The Ultimate Potato Book

The Ultimate Brownie Book

The Ultimate Shrimp Book

The ULTIMATE MUFFIN Book

More Than 600 Recipes for Sweet and Savory Muffins

Bruce Weinstein and Mark Scarbrough

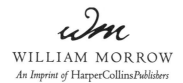

WILLIAM MORROW

An Imprint of HarperCollinsPublishers

HarperCollins books may be purchased for educational, business, or sales promotional use. For information please write: Special Markets Department, HarperCollins Publishers Inc., 10 East 53rd Street, New York, NY 10022.

FIRST EDITION

Designed by Renato Stanisic

Printed on acid-free paper

Library of Congress Cataloging-in-Publication Data

Weinstein, Bruce, 1960–
    The ultimate muffin book / Bruce Weinstein and Mark Scarbrough.
        p.   cm.
    Includes bibliographical references and index.
    ISBN 0-06-009676-4 (pbk.)
    1. Muffins.   I. Scarbrough, Mark.   II. Title.

TX770.M83.W45   2004
641.8'157—dc22   2003059273

08   WBC/QW   10   9   8   7   6   5   4

Front Cover Recipe: Lemonade Muffins
Back Cover Recipe: Berry Muffins

To Pat Adrian

A darn good dinner companion, an even better friend

Contents

Acknowledgments

First and foremost, a huge "hurrah!" for Harriet Bell, ever the guru, ever the friend: a whiz at editing, sales, imagination, everything her job demands. We're just flat lucky she's our editor.

Many kudos to Susan Ginsburg at Writers House. She does exactly what an agent's supposed to do: negotiates, says "no," says "yes," says "maybe," and all around encourages us to do our best work, even the day after her blowout birthday party.

Hats off to Lucy Baker at Morrow—new to the job yet on top of her game. Thanks for making this book so easy.

The same to Rachel Spector at Writers House. She answered queries quickly, dealt with problems, trivial and stupendous—and, most important, still knows how to laugh off writerly neuroses.

This book wouldn't have happened without Pat Adrian's encouragement and advice—no wonder it's dedicated to her. What's more, she's game to order absolutely anything with us in the culinary empyrean of New York City.

Beth Shepard continues to man the fires of publicity—and we can't thank her enough for her work, her energy, and her "hey, what's the big deal?" attitude.

And a big shout-out to our favorite pro, Juli Vitello, who's willing to let us do just about whatever we want on CN8's "Your Morning" (within reason, of course).

Thanks, once again, to Carrie Weinberg, Gypsy Lovett, and Bobbilynn Jones at HarperCollins for getting the word out—and for being willing to try new things in a very crowded market.

Thanks to Petra Hoy for copyediting the manuscript and making our job so much simpler once the manuscript went in. Thanks to Renato Stanisic for designing such a readable book. And once again, as ever, thanks to Quentin Bacon for a great cover shot.

A big cheer for Ann Cahn, the most unsung hero at HarperCollins. We can breathe easily when someone so competent has her hand on production editorial's rudder.

Who knew the members of the Stonewall Chorale could eat so many muffins? Thanks for plowing through the test batches and being willing to take home whatever we brought to rehearsal.

The ULTIMATE
MUFFIN *Book*

Introduction

Picture this: a gathering of black-bedecked New Yorkers after work, sipping drinks, talking in murmurs. We walk in, exhausted from testing recipes, laden with cake boxes. Heads turn. From behind minuscule glasses, someone asks, "What'd *you* bring?" We duck our heads—was this really the right thing to bring to a techno-urban wasteland of the terminally hip?—and say, "We made muffins." Bingo. Everyone smiles. They grab the boxes, tear them open, laugh, enjoy themselves.

And not once, but over and over again this scenario played out as we were testing recipes. Why do muffins inspire such unbounded delight? Is it their taste? Their homeyness? Their simplicity? Whatever it is, it's irresistible, even in Manhattan.

The story of muffins is something of a mystery. Nothing nefarious, of course, just murky. Most homespun treats (think here of brownies or gingerbread) have hard-to-discover origins; any lapse in their histories is prone to sheer guess.

Some food writers consider the "American" muffin to be the kissing cousin of the English muffin, that fork-separated, disk-like, yeast-raised bread popularized by Samuel B. Thomas, a Boston baker of British extraction. But here's the rub, the one those descriptors should automatically have given away: "fork-separated," "disk-like," and "yeast-raised" are the very things an American muffin isn't. We can safely say that the only thing English muffins and American muffins have in common is a name, *muffin*.

Many claim the word *muffin* is derived from *muff*, as in *a little muff*, or a small hand warmer. So people walked around clutching warm bread on winter days? Not likely. As Laura Mason points out in *The Oxford Companion to Food*, *muffin* is another culinary term borrowed from France, this time the archaic word *moufflet*, or soft, a reference to the irresistible texture of warm bread.

Admittedly, the first muffins baked in the New World were hardly irresistible. They were plain, even excessively so, varied only by the flour used: graham, wheat, rye, flax, or oat. But even such grim-faced, eat-your-prunes alterations indicated there was already variability in the recipes. As one deviation lead to another, it's easy to see how we got to the stunning array of muffins available today—especially since muffins are so easy to make.

An enduring American passion for doing things fast also contributes to their popularity. Muffins are quick breads—that is, breads that rise thanks to a speedy chemical reaction, rather than through the far slower organic action of yeast. Most likely, we've all done that junior high chemistry experiment of mixing baking soda (an alkali, sometimes called a base) with vinegar (an acid) to create a bubbly volcano of carbon dioxide froth. If not, there's no time like the present. Pour 1/4 cup vinegar into a tall glass and place it in the sink. Stir in 1 teaspoon baking soda and watch it go. When those bubbles get to work in a quick bread batter, they don't fritter away into nothing. They're stabilized (or trapped) by the flour's glutens. And voilà, a fast and easy stand-in for yeast.

Despite our passion for speed, quick breads were not quick to catch on. They were an innovation of the late 1700s that took almost two centuries to bear fruit. That's partly because baking soda was not the original leavener. That distinction goes to pearl ash (or potassium carbonate), a compound whose manufacturing process was patented by Samuel Hopkins on July 31, 1790. The making of pearl ash was a frugal venture, replete with Yankee ingenuity. It started with wood ashes, a household annoyance in colonial America. Hopkins took the ashes and soaked them in warm water in a one to ten ratio for twenty-four hours. The sediment was discarded; the resulting liquid was gray, viscous, and most likely carcinogenic. It was boiled down to produce an opaque, whitish residue, aka *pearl* ash, which produced that chemical froth of carbon dioxide when mixed with an acid and liquids (or acidic liquids, like soured milk, something housewives had in abundance before modern refrigeration).

Although a boon to bakers who could forgo the tedium of yeast, pearl ash never really caught on because it had the unfortunate side effect of creating soap when combined with fats like butter or lard—not exactly a taste sensation. But if not pearl ash, the thinking went, then surely something else would make bread fast, thanks to a similar chemical process.

The answer was found in nineteenth-century druggists' pantries: sodium bicarbonate, now known as "baking soda." This digestive aid could be used in the same way as pearl ash—that is, in the presence of an acid and a liquid—but with almost no soapy aftertaste. And it had homeopathic properties, to boot.

By the 1830s, American homemakers were heading off to their pharmacists for their baking needs. But why only use soured milk, which gives breads a certain whang. Why not use fresh milk? That would require acid in another form, a powdered form. And while we're at it, why wait to put the alkali and acid together? If they need moisture to interact, why not put them together in a dry compound in advance?

American druggists were quick to sniff the winds of profitability—and they were soon combining sodium bicarbonate with another low-grade acid found on their shelves: cream of tartar. This is the acidic residue scraped out of wine casks after production; it was used at the time for a variety of health complaints. The resulting compound of baking soda and cream of tartar could be kept dry with a little corn starch to absorb any excess moisture.

But what about cream of tartar? Isn't that associated with wine? Mustn't it be, in Victorian terms, wicked? So—ever depressingly so—there arose a small industry of preachers and health reformers decrying 1) the lazy women who would want to forgo the rigors of yeast, and 2) their devilish helper in this indolence, this new-fangled leavener from wine.

In 1859, a fast-thinking Boston entrepreneur, Eben Norton Horsford, patented his answer: sodium bicarbonate and a different acid, calcium phosphate. He called his product "Horsford's Cream of Tartar Substitute." The name proved unwieldy—and unmarketable—so he repackaged it as "Rumford Baking Powder," named for the professorship Horsford held at Harvard, the Rumford Chair of the Application of Science to the Useful Arts, but also named as a kind of elixir, a "powder," like the other ones created during antebellum America (headache powders and the like), powders that could get the job done quickly, almost magically.

Now home cooks were whipping up batters without a yeast worry—except that the new baking powder worked too well. It reacted so quickly in the presence of liquids that any leavening was over by the time the batter hit the oven. So there was one final chapter in this story: in 1889, double-acting baking powder came along. A second acidic leavening agent was added to the mixture, an acid that reacted slowly in the presence of moisture, but quickly once heat was added—thus, "double-acting": once with liquid, and again with heat.

And so you may think, with the quick-bread revolution under way, it was a short trip to the muffin's cultural ascendancy, right?

Not so. There's no mention of muffins in late nineteenth-century cookbooks. There's not a single reference to muffins in any Boston Cooking School cookbook until 1923, eight years after Fanny Farmer's death. And there's not one reference to muffins on American menus archived in the New York Public Library from the 1920s and '30s.

One problem may have been muffins' homespun nature. They're hardly the stuff of Parisian or Swiss bakers, and certainly not the highbrow confections that were increasingly the staples of East and West coast enclaves during the Jazz Age of the twentieth century.

Furthermore, muffins were originally not as sweet as we might imagine. One of the first muffin crazes came out of Battle Creek, Michigan, home of Dr. John Harvey Kellogg's Seventh Day Adventist health camp and soon-to-be cereal factory. Bran muffins, of course, were among Kellogg's many obsessions, both gastric and financial. He could sell more bran cereal by making it a necessary ingredient in recipes. Through his efforts, the muffin gained a reputation around 1920 as a kind of speedy purgative you could whip up every morning. Echoes of that heritage still trail muffins. It's amazing how many people think they're eating something healthy, despite the splendid combination of butter, sugar, and flour.

But healthy eating has never been a longlasting trend. Soon enough, the world wars were over; the Depression, a memory. Butter was no longer rationed. Muffin tins became nonstick; ovens, more conventional. Convenience reigned supreme.

And so muffins were on their way to utter excess. Ever-more-affluent Americans developed a taste for sweeter, richer treats, more like cake than bread. Bed-and-breakfasts and country inns undoubtedly spurred this fad along. Their chefs gave their citified patrons a light but high-fat dessert, even at breakfast.

Far be it from us to turn puritanical at the end of this story, but in the last decades of the twentieth century we've witnessed what we call the "cupcakeization" of muffins. Yes, to be palatable, muffins needed more sugar and fat, all Kellogg's assertions about dry bran notwithstanding—but they certainly didn't need the poundage under which some now labor.

It's not that we're fussy about sugar and butter. We did write *The Ultimate Brownie Book*, after all. Simply put, muffins aren't cakes. They're quick breads; they should have a breadlike texture. To that end, we've honored their down-home roots by using a variety of flavors, whole wheat and oat to name two of the most common in our recipes. And we've cut down the sugar. Don't worry—the muffins are still sweet. Some, very sweet— just try the Fudge or Honey Muffins. But most are less sugary, more flavorful, and good for breakfast, lunch, or dinner.

We've also included savory muffins, ones a tad unexpected to some. These veer farthest from the cupcake trend—Potato or Quiche Lorraine Muffins, for example. Any of these would make a nice accompaniment to a roast, a baked ham, or a Thanksgiving turkey. Think of them not just as bread, but as a side dish.

All that said, there are points where we're less persnickety than some bakers. Some cookbooks stipulate what muffins should look like (in some cases, the exact angle of their peaks), or how they should feel when broken open. But what makes a muffin, by definition, is its shape from the tin and the quick bread technique used to create it. Just as we're not wedded to one taste, we're also not wedded to one texture. Muffins should be breadlike, yes—but there's a world of latitude. So you'll find a variety of textures in this book, just as you do when you walk into your local bake shop. Some are flat-topped; others are conical, even cracked. Some poof out like mushrooms; others widen out along the sides. Some specialty muffins—like Angel Food Muffins—don't rise at all.

It's a matter of which texture, or crumb, works best for what's in the batter. Our preferences? We like a moister fruit muffin, a good platform for tart berries or sliced peaches; but we like a drier cocoa muffin, one that's slightly heavier, denser, providing an intense taste of chocolate that's not watered down.

And while we're on the matter of preferences, there are a few omissions in this book. Yeast muffins, for one. We didn't feel they had any place in a book which celebrates America's favorite quick bread. Nor did we include a recipe simply because it could be baked or molded in a muffin tin, like meatloaf muffins or chicken salad muffins.

Omissions aside, there are hundreds of muffins here, from Lemon to Apple, Margarita to Daiquiri. You'll find this variety presented alphabetically: Almond, Angel Food, Apple, Applesauce, Apricot, and so on.

Each recipe is followed by a series of variations, usually made with one addition to the batter, or one substitution. Here's where we get creative—or go crazy, depending on your perspective. Pumpkin Muffins are all well and good, perfect for jam or jelly. But then there's Cranberry Pumpkin Muffins, Marshmallow Nut Pumpkin Muffins, Orange Pecan Pumpkin Muffins, Pumpkin Seed Pumpkin Muffins, and Spiced Pumpkin Muffins. That's enough variety to last us all a good long while, and certainly enough muffins to make everyone we know smile.

Making Muffins

TIPS FOR SUCCESSFUL MUFFINS

1. Check the weather.
Odd, yes, but quick breads suffer under high humidity, which causes the batter to turn sticky and glutinous. If the day's particularly damp, reduce the amount of liquid in the batter just slightly. If the recipe calls for 1/2 cup of milk, fill the measuring cup to just shy of the rim, thereby reducing the amount of liquid in the batter by perhaps 1 tablespoon and giving the day's humidity its due.

2. Preheat the oven.
Muffins need a hot oven to rise properly. Preheat yours for 15 minutes, time enough to collect the ingredients and whip up the batter.

3. Cool the melted butter.
Hot melted butter can shock both the flour's glutens and the leavening agent, reducing the rise in the muffins. It can also lead to bits of scrambled egg in the batter. So give the melted butter about 5 minutes to cool down.

4. Let the eggs come to room temperature.
Cold eggs can shock the leavening and retard the poof of the muffin's famous hat. If you leave the eggs in their shell on the counter for about 15 minutes, they'll be just right. If you're in a hurry, place them in a bowl of room temperature water for 5 minutes before cracking them.

5. If you want, beat the egg whites separately and fold them in later.
As we were testing recipes, we went back and forth on this one—should we make it a standard rule or not? We finally decided it was too much for a book about a down-home treat. Still, for some recipes, like Chocolate Chip Muffins, we've held to this fussier technique simply to lighten a batter weighed down with, say, chocolate chips. You can do the same for any sweet muffin. (We don't recommend this technique for savory muffins—these should be denser and chewier.) Add the yolks where it indicates to add the eggs, then beat the egg whites separately in a medium bowl with an electric mixer at high speed, until soft peaks form. Fold the beaten whites into the batter after you've added the dry ingredients. It's a sure way to make very light, tender muffins.

6. Mix the dry ingredients in a separate bowl.
The salt and leavening need to be evenly distributed throughout the flour before the mixture is added to the wet ingredients. This ensures the proper rise and texture once the muffins are baked.

7. Don't sift the flour.
You're making a quick bread, not a cake. For the best crumb, spoon the flour into a measuring cup, then level it off with the back of the spoon.

8. Unless it's specifically called for, leave the electric mixer in the cabinet.
An electric mixer will set the flour's glutens too stiff. Use a whisk to beat the eggs, then a wooden spoon to mix in the dry ingredients. Whatever you do, don't overmix—stir only until the flour is moistened. As with pancake batter, leave the lumps alone.

9. Wash the muffin tins before you fill them.
Dry the individual cups carefully on the top and in the indentations, but don't dry the bottom of the entire muffin pan. The remaining moisture will produce a little steam in the oven, which will crisp the muffin tops as they rise, much as you might spritz the oven with water as you bake bread for a crunchier crust.

10. Grease the muffin tins, even if they're nonstick.

A layer of fat between the batter and the tin does three things: 1) it protects the batter from super-heating in the oven, 2) it allows the sides to crisp, and 3) it makes clean-up a snap. We recommend using a nonstick spray, even one with added flour, like Baker's Joy. You can also use butter—or the wrapper it came in, so long as it has some soft butter still adhering to it.

11. Fill the muffin cups three-quarters full.

Leave enough room for the muffins to expand as they bake. And don't press down when you fill the tins. The batter will naturally collapse in the oven's heat. If you have extra batter, either place it in extra tins or in individual, oven-safe, 1/2-cup, greased ramekins, or reserve the batter for a second baking. If you've used double-acting baking powder, it should be allright—the muffins won't be as light as those from the first baking, but they'll still be moist and tender.

12. Fill any unused muffin cups with water.

Doing so will help the nearby muffins bake evenly; it will also keep those near the empty indention from drying out. Plus, the added water will keep metal tins from warping under the oven's high heat.

13. Work quickly.

You can, of course, prepare the wet and dry ingredients separately, then take a break, perhaps to prepare the rest of the meal (although don't let the egg mixture sit at room temperature for more than 30 minutes). But don't dally once you've combined the wet and dry ingredients; spoon the batter into the tins and bake the muffins right away.

14. Treat baking times as guides, not law.

Even modern ovens have hot spots. Some have temperature swings, thanks to less-sensitive thermostats. And sometimes the density of one brand of flour over another or variants in the size of a "large" egg are enough to throw off the baking times slightly. Always check for doneness with a metal cake tester or a toothpick, as directed in the recipes.

15. Don't be quick to unmold the muffins.

Once the tins are out of the oven, cool them on wire racks for at least 5 minutes, or sometimes longer for more delicate muffins. For the best structure, muffins need to let off steam in their tins, condensing slightly with the form holding them intact.

16. Rewarm muffins in their tins.

Tip them up, so that their tops are at an angle, one corner of the bottom still touching the tin. Then place them in a warm (but off) oven for about 5 minutes.

17. Thaw muffins at room temperature.

Most muffins freeze exceptionally well. The exceptions are those with fresh berries and stone fruits, often found among the variations in this book—the problem is not freezing, of course, but thawing: too much moisture ruins the crumb. These are best simply stored at room temperature. To freeze the rest of the muffins presented here, seal them, once they're cool, in a freezer-safe bag and store the muffins in the freezer as indicated in the recipe. To serve, let them stand at room temperature for at least 2 hours, or for 4 hours if they contain any fruit. We don't recommend heating them after they've been frozen—minuscule ice crystals in the muffins will melt and then steam, thereby compromising the texture by turning them gummy.

A WORD ABOUT MUFFIN TINS

One warning: there is no standard size. The base recipes here were developed to make 12 muffins from a tin in which each indention, when full, holds 1/2 cup water. Some of the variations will make up to 18 such muffins.

Your tins may be smaller or slightly larger. If your tin is smaller, you'll need to shave two or three minutes off the baking time. If yours is larger, you'll need to add a few minutes. Always check for doneness with a toothpick or a metal cake tester, as indicated in the recipe.

Silicon muffin tins must be placed on a baking sheet before being placed in the oven. For best results, use an insulated baking sheet, one with a small layer of air trapped between the metal sheets.

From any of these recipes, you can also make mini muffins or extra-large ones, depending on the shape of your tins; however, the baking times will vary significantly. As a rough rule of thumb, figure on about half the time for mini muffins, and about one-third additional time for the extra-large ones. You can also use the tins that make only so-called muffin tops, although we recommend baking sweet and cakey muffins in them, like the Honey, Walnut, or Sesame, and not using this specialty tin for any of the savory muffins or either of the Angel Food muffins. Muffin tops, exposed to so much heat so fast, bake very quickly—in about two-thirds of the baking time indicated in the recipe—so watch them closely.

A GUIDE TO SOME INGREDIENTS

Baking Powder

Keep it dry at all costs, and use only double-acting baking powder because muffins need all the help they can get—they must double or even triple in size in a matter of minutes.

Baking powder, even kept dry, loses its efficacy over time as the acid and alkali slowly react, any added cornstarch to absorb moisture notwithstanding. As a rule, replace baking powder after three months. To check if yours is viable, dissolve 1 teaspoon in 1 cup of water. If it bubbles vigorously, you're good to go.

If you're concerned about chemical additives in various brands of baking powder, you can make your own by whisking together 1/3 cup cream of tartar, 3 tablespoons baking soda, and 1 1/2 tablespoons cornstarch in a clean, dry, medium bowl. Sift the mixture twice through a fine-mesh sieve or a chinoise, then place it in a pot or jar, seal tightly, and store at room temperature for up to three months in a dark, dry place. One warning: this is single-acting baking powder, not double-acting—so use all the batter you make in a single round of baking.

Baking Soda

Baking soda also loses its efficacy over time. Make sure yours is kept scrupulously dry. Even so, replace it after three months. Never use baking soda that's been stored in the refrigerator to trap food odors.

Bran

Bran is made from the outer shell or husk from one of several grains. The husks are usually removed in the milling process. To make bran, they're ground to a fine powder which is high in fiber, calcium, and phosphorus. For more tooth in any sweet muffin, replace 2 tablespoons all-purpose flour with 2 tablespoons wheat bran.

Oat bran is, obviously enough, the ground hulls of oats, and a great source of soluble fiber. It adds a silky texture to muffins, but is very heavy and needs to be lightened in a batter, usually with beaten egg whites.

Butter

Our recipes call for unsalted butter, the baking standard.

We have not used solid vegetable shortening in any recipe—although you may want to if you want muffins that have a crumb closer to bakeshop varieties. Use only half the butter indicated; substitute an equivalent amount of solid vegetable shortening for the missing butter. Melt both together and cool before proceeding with the recipe.

If you melt butter in a microwave, beware of the splatter effect, caused by the butter melting on the inside, then superheating and bursting out of the sides. To prevent this, cut the butter into 1 tablespoon sections, place them in a small bowl, and microwave in 15 second increments, swirling the bowl after each heating. When almost all the butter is melted, remove the bowl from the microwave and let the residual heat melt any remainder.

Buttermilk

Although low-fat (or 1 percent) buttermilk will produce consistently good muffins, do not use nonfat buttermilk.

Buttermilk is one baking staple most of us don't keep on hand. One solution is to substitute powdered buttermilk, often available in gourmet markets and specialty food stores. Simply make the amount of buttermilk you need, based on the package's instructions, then add it to the batter as indicated.

Cocoa Nibs

The quintessence of chocolate, these are coarsely ground roasted cocoa beans. They add a crunchy, nutty taste to any batter. Store them sealed at room temperature for up to six months.

Cocoa Powder

To make cocoa powder, the cocoa butter is mostly extracted from cocoa; the resulting solids (called chocolate liquor) are dried, then ground to a powder.

Cocoa powder is available in two forms: regular (sometimes called natural) and Dutch-processed, which has been treated with an alkali to neutralize chocolate's natural acidity.

Always sift cocoa powder; any clumps will not be beaten out in the few seconds it takes for the muffin batter to come together.

Coconut

Coconut flakes are available in two forms: 1) sweetened, sold in the baking aisle of most supermarkets, and 2) unsweetened, usually available at health food markets or at some gourmet stores in the bulk food section. These recipes call for each on different occasions; use only the kind called for in the recipe. To store, seal tightly in plastic bags for up to six months.

Coconut milk is made from cooking coconut flesh in water, then straining out the solids. The resulting "milk" is thick and luxurious. From the can, it should be stirred before adding it to a batter.

Light coconut milk is actually just the second pressing of the same solids used in the making of coconut milk. The resulting milk has less fat, is thinner, and has a less intense taste—although it is healthier for you.

Cream of coconut is a sweetened concoction best used for frozen drinks—and very sweet muffins. Use it only when called for; never substitute cream of coconut for coconut milk or vice versa.

Dried Bananas

Dried bananas are long and thin, like bananas themselves, and so should be chopped before using. Those found in health food stores and gourmet markets are often dark brown because they lack preservatives. Don't confuse them with fried banana chips, which are too oily for successful baking.

Flour

For these recipes, use all-purpose flour, preferably unbleached. If you store flour in the refrigerator, let it come to room temperature before using.

As we developed these recipes, we discovered that muffins benefit from a variety of flours. Here are several "alternative flours" called for:

Oat Flour Made from ground oats, this adds a velvety texture when combined with wheat flour. For the best taste, look for brands made from whole grains.

Rice Flour Made from ground white or brown rice, this common flour substitute is gluten-free. Do not substitute glutinous rice flour, which is used almost exclusively in Asian confectionery.

Spelt Flour A cereal grain with a light but nutty taste, spelt is not gluten-free, but it sometimes can be tolerated by those with wheat allergies. It has a very high protein content.

Tapioca Flour Made from the ground root of the cassava plant, tapioca is an ancient thickener, used in Asia much as Westerners have used corn starch. Gluten-free, it should be combined with other flours, like rice flour, for the best results.

Maple Sugar

This highly sweet sugar is made by boiling maple sap down past the syrup stage, until it crystallizes into coarse grains. It is available in gourmet markets and specialty food stores.

Maple Syrup

Maple syrup is packaged in the United States in two grades: A and B. Grade B is often used for baking, but we find it too pungent for muffins. Grade A comes in three varieties: Light Amber, Medium Amber, and Dark Amber. The first two, while great for pancakes, are lost in baking, so use Grade A Dark Amber, if possible. It's assertive without the whang of Grade B.

Marzipan

A mixture of ground almonds, sugar, and sometimes glycerin or egg whites, marzipan can be beaten into muffin batters, provided it's soft and pliable, not hard and dusty. If the marzipan is hard, soften it in the microwave for 15 seconds on high. One warning: this produces mixed results, especially if the almond oil heats and falls out of suspension, creating a greasy mess. To avoid this problem, check to make sure the marzipan you're buying in the baking aisle is fresh and soft.

Milk

In most recipes where milk is used, we've given you a choice among whole, low-fat, or nonfat. Thus, you can make anything from a full-fat to a relatively healthy muffin, depending on what you want. In some recipes, however, we've indicated you shouldn't use nonfat milk. In these, the extra fat, even the small amount in low-fat milk, will keep the muffins moister than they would be with nonfat milk.

Nut Oils

Pressed from nuts like almonds, walnuts, or hazelnuts, nut oils are excellent in quick breads, lending a good flavor and a lighter texture when compared to muffins made with butter. Store nut oils in the refrigerator for up to three months. They go rancid quickly, so check to make sure the oil still has a bright, fresh, nutty aroma before using.

Parmigiano-Reggiano

There is no substitute for this hard, skimmed cow's milk Italian cheese. Grate it into batters using a cheese grater or the small holes of a box grater. Buy small chunks, cut from larger wheels, with as little rind as possible to cut down on any waste. Do not use canned, imitation Parmesan cheese which is made mostly from oil and preservatives.

Sugar

Use granulated sugar unless otherwise indicated.

Most of the time, the sugar is mixed with the flour, not first dissolved into the wet ingredients. (The one exception is brown sugar, which will clump in the dry ingredients.) Muffins are slightly denser and have a better crumb if the sugar is not whipped with the eggs, as it would be in a cake batter.

Vanilla Extract

If possible, use pure vanilla extract, not an imitation flavoring. A double-strength extract, such as that available from Penzeys Spices (see Source Guide, page 237), will add even more flavor.

If you ever make a recipe that calls for whole vanilla beans, don't throw out the pods if you have merely scraped the seeds out of them. Cut the pods into small sections and add them to your bottle of vanilla extract for a more intense flavor.

Yogurt

Use only plain yogurt, unless otherwise indicated; but you may use regular, low-fat, or nonfat, based on your preference.

A Note About High-Altitude Baking

For baking muffins at altitudes from 3,000 to 5,000 feet above sea level, decrease the baking powder by ⅛ teaspoon, decrease the sugar by 1 teaspoon per ½ cup used, and add 1 tablespoon more liquid to the batter (milk, if used, or water, if no milk is used).

Above 5,000 feet, decrease the baking powder by ¼ teaspoon, decrease the sugar by 1 tablespoon per ½ cup used, and increase the liquid by 3 tablespoons. Also increase the oven temperature by 10°F.

Muffin Recipes A to Z

Almond Muffins

Makes 12 muffins

Almond oil is rich in omega-9 acids and so is a heart-healthy alternative to other fats. But almond oil can also produce gummy muffins. Here, a small amount of butter is combined with the aromatic oil for a lighter crumb with that characteristic, nutty flavor. Almond oil is found in almost all gourmet markets and in some supermarkets in the cooking oil section. Store it in the refrigerator, but let it come to room temperature before using it in this recipe.

Nonstick spray or paper muffin cups
3/4 cup sliced blanched almonds
2 cups all-purpose flour
1/2 cup sugar
1 tablespoon baking powder
1/2 teaspoon salt
1 large egg, at room temperature
3/4 cup milk (whole, low-fat, or nonfat)
2 tablespoons honey
1/2 teaspoon vanilla extract
1/2 teaspoon almond extract
1/4 cup almond oil
3 tablespoons unsalted butter, melted and cooled

1. Position the rack in the center of the oven and preheat the oven to 400°F. To prepare the muffin tins, spray the indentations and the rims around them with nonstick spray, or line the indentations with paper muffin cups. If using silicon muffin tins, spray as directed, then place them on a baking sheet.

2. Spread the almonds out on a second cookie sheet and toast for about 5 minutes, or until golden and fragrant, stirring occasionally. Transfer the nuts to a large plate and cool for 5 minutes.

3. Pour 1/2 cup of the toasted almonds into a mini food processor or wide-base blender; pulse 5 or 6 times until finely ground. Be careful not to grind the nuts to a paste. Transfer the ground nuts to a medium bowl; stir in the flour, sugar, baking powder, and salt until well combined. Set aside.

4. Whisk the egg, milk, honey, and vanilla and almond extracts in a large bowl until smooth and thick, about 1 minute, then whisk in the oil and butter until well combined. Using a wooden spoon, stir in the remaining 1/4 cup sliced almonds and the flour mixture just until the dry ingredients are moistened.

5. Fill the prepared tins three-quarters full. Use additional greased tins or small, oven-safe, greased ramekins for any leftover batter, or reserve the batter for a second baking. Bake for 20 minutes, or until the muffins are golden brown with rounded, cracked tops. A toothpick inserted into the center of one muffin should come out with a few moist crumbs attached.

6. Set the pan on a wire rack to cool for 10 minutes. Gently tip each muffin to one side to make sure it isn't stuck. If one is, gently rock it back and forth to release it. Remove the muffins from the pan and cool them for 5 minutes more on the rack before serving. If storing or freezing the muffins, cool them completely before sealing in an airtight container or freezer-safe plastic bags. The muffins will stay fresh for up to 24 hours at room temperature or up to 2 months in the freezer.

Almond Apple Poppy Seed Muffins: *Add 1/2 cup chopped dried apple and 2 tablespsoons poppy seeds with the almond oil.*

Almond Blueberry Muffins: *Sprinkle 6 fresh blueberries onto the top of each muffin before baking. You will need 1/2 pint of blueberries.*

Almond Cranberry Muffins: *Add 1/2 cup dried cranberries with the flour.*

Almond Date Muffins: *Add 1/2 cup chopped, pitted dates with the flour.*

Almond Joy Muffins: *Add 1/4 cup sweetened shredded coconut and 1/4 cup mini chocolate chips with the flour.*

Almond Nut Crunch Muffins: *Top the muffins with Nut Crunch Topping (page 229) before baking.*

Almond Streusel Muffins: *Top the muffins with Cinnamon Streusel Topping (page 224) or Low-Fat Streusel Topping (page 228) before baking.*

Angel Food Muffins

Makes 12 muffins

Like angel food cake, these muffins are best with tea after dinner, or with a glass of milk before bed. They're light and airy because beaten egg whites are the only leavening. You'll get the most volume out of the whites if you beat them when they're at room temperature. Make sure that the mixing bowl is at room temperature and that there's not a drop of yolk, grease, or water with the whites before you beat them.

Nonstick spray
1 cup cake or all-purpose flour, plus additional for the muffin tins
1 cup sugar
8 large egg whites, at room temperature
$^1/_2$ teaspoon salt
1 teaspoon cream of tartar
2 teaspoons vanilla extract

1. Position the rack in the center of the oven and preheat the oven to 350°F. To prepare the muffin tins, spray the indentations and the rims around them with nonstick spray. Sprinkle a pinch of flour into each of the indentations and shake the tin around, rapping your hands on the bottom and sides to coat the interior surface of the muffin cups with flour. Shake out any excess flour by rapping the tin against the side of the sink. If using silicon muffin tins, forgo dusting them with flour—simply spray the tins and place them on a baking sheet.

2. Whisk 1 cup flour with 1/2 cup sugar in a medium bowl until blended. Set aside.

3. In a large bowl, beat the egg whites and salt with an electric mixer at medium speed until foamy, about 1 minute. Raise the speed to high, beat in the cream of tartar, and continue beating until soft peaks form. With the mixer running, add the remaining 1/2 cup sugar in a slow stream, then beat in the vanilla. Continue beating for about 3 minutes, or until the mixture is stiff and shiny and until no sugar granules can be felt when a bit of beaten egg white is rubbed between your fingertips.

4. Use a rubber spatula to fold in a third of the flour mixture. Do not beat; fold in long, even arcs, so that the whites stay fluffy but the flour is evenly distributed. Fold in half of the remaining flour mixture using the same technique. Then very gently

fold in the remaining flour mixture, just so that the flour is mixed in, but not so that it dissolves.

5. Fill the prepared tins to the top; divide any remaining batter equally among the tins, piling it as high above the rims as necessary. Bake for 28 minutes, or until well browned.

6. Place the tins on a wire rack to cool for 45 minutes. Gently rock the muffins back and forth to release them from the tins. Store the muffins in an airtight container at room temperature for 24 hours or freeze them in freezer-safe bags for up to 2 months.

> **Cinnamon Angel Food Muffins:** *Add 1 1/2 teaspoons ground cinnamon with the flour.*
>
> **Lemon Angel Food Muffins:** *Add 2 teaspoons grated lemon zest and 1 teaspoon lemon extract with the vanilla. If desired, drizzle the cooled muffins with Lemon Drizzle (page 227).*
>
> **Orange Angel Food Muffins:** *Add 2 teaspoons grated orange zest and 1 teaspoon orange extract with the vanilla.*
>
> **Rose Angel Food Muffins:** *Add 2 teaspoons rose water with the vanilla.*
>
> **Vanilla Glazed Angel Food Muffins:** *Coat the cooled muffins with Vanilla Dip (page 231).*

Apple Muffins

Makes 12 muffins

This recipe is adapted from Bruce's grandmother's dairy-free apple cake, often served for dessert on Friday nights. The apples are first macerated in sugar and oil. The result is an incredibly moist batter—and one well-suited to muffins. One warning: the muffins don't brown, so bake them only until a toothpick or cake tester comes out almost clean.

> **3 medium Granny Smith apples, peeled, cored, and diced**
> **1 cup sugar**
> **$^1/_2$ cup canola or vegetable oil**
> **Nonstick spray or paper muffin cups**
> **$2^1/_4$ cups all-purpose flour**
> **1 tablespoon baking powder**
> **$^1/_2$ teaspoon salt**
> **$^1/_4$ teaspoon ground cinnamon**
> **$^1/_4$ teaspoon grated nutmeg**
> **$^1/_2$ cup milk (whole, low-fat, or nonfat)**
> **1 large egg, lightly beaten, at room temperature**

1. Toss the diced apples with the sugar in a medium bowl. Pour the oil over the top, stir well, and set aside at room temperature for 45 minutes.

2. Position the rack in the center of the oven and preheat the oven to 400°F. To prepare the muffin tins, spray the indentations and the rims around them with nonstick spray, or line the indentations with paper muffin cups. If using silicon muffin tins, spray as directed, then place them on a baking sheet.

3. Whisk the flour, baking powder, salt, cinnamon, and nutmeg in a second medium bowl until uniform. Set aside.

4. Using a wooden spoon, stir the milk and egg into the apple mixture until smooth. Then stir in the prepared flour mixture until moistened.

5. Fill the prepared tins three-quarters full. Use additional greased tins or small, oven-safe, greased ramekins for any leftover batter, or reserve the batter for a second baking. Bake for 25 minutes, or until the muffins have rounded, slightly cracked tops. A

toothpick inserted in the center of one muffin should come out with just a few moist crumbs attached.

6. Set the pan on a wire rack to cool for 10 minutes. Gently rock the muffins back and forth to release them from the tins. Remove them from the pan and cool them for 5 minutes more on the rack before serving. If storing or freezing the muffins, cool them completely before sealing in an airtight container or freezer-safe plastic bags. The muffins will stay fresh for up to 48 hours at room temperature or up to 2 months in the freezer.

Apple Cheddar Muffins: *Sprinkle each muffin with 1 tablespoon shredded Cheddar before baking. You'll need 3/4 cup shredded cheese.*

Apple Cherry Muffins: *Stir 3/4 cup dried cherries into the diced apples before adding the sugar and the oil.*

Apple Cranberry Muffins: *Stir 3/4 cup chopped fresh cranberries into the diced apples before adding the sugar and the oil.*

Apple Crumb Muffins: *Sprinkle the top of muffins with Crumb Topping (page 226) before baking.*

Apple Pecan Muffins: *Add 3/4 cup chopped pecans with the flour.*

Apple Raisin Muffins: *Stir 3/4 cup dark raisins into the diced apples before adding the sugar and the oil.*

Applesauce Muffins

Makes 12 muffins

The taste says apple pie, the crumb says apple cake, but the shape says muffin. Everyone who tries them will just say, "More." Although the recipe calls for unsweetened applesauce, you can vary the batter with any of the unsweetened fruit and applesauce combinations available in your market.

Nonstick spray or paper muffin cups
2 cups all-purpose flour
2 tablespoons granulated sugar
2 teaspoons baking powder
1 teaspoon baking soda
1/2 teaspoon salt
1/2 teaspoon ground cinnamon
1 large egg, at room temperature
1/2 cup packed light brown sugar
1 1/4 cups unsweetened applesauce
6 tablespoons (3/4 stick) unsalted butter, melted and cooled
1/4 cup milk (whole, low-fat, or nonfat)

1. Position the rack in the center of the oven and preheat the oven to 400°F. To prepare the muffin tins, spray the indentations and the rims around them with nonstick spray, or line the indentations with paper muffin cups. If using silicon muffin tins, spray as directed, then place them on a baking sheet.

2. Whisk the flour, granulated sugar, baking powder, baking soda, salt, and cinnamon in a medium bowl until uniform. Set aside.

3. In a second medium bowl, whisk the egg and brown sugar for 3 minutes, or until thick and pale brown. Whisk in the applesauce, melted butter, and milk, until blended. Using a wooden spoon, stir in the prepared flour mixture until moistened.

4. Fill the prepared tins three-quarters full. Use additional greased tins or small, oven-safe, greased ramekins for any leftover batter, or reserve the batter for a second baking. Bake for 20 minutes, or until the muffins are lightly browned with rounded

tops. A toothpick inserted into the center of one muffin should come out fairly clean, with a crumb or two attached.

5. Set the pan on a wire rack to cool for 10 minutes. Gently rock each muffin back and forth to release it. Remove the muffins from the pan and cool them for 5 minutes more on the rack before serving. If storing or freezing the muffins, cool completely before sealing them in an airtight container or freezer-safe plastic bags. The muffins will stay fresh for up to 2 days at room temperature, or up to 2 months in the freezer.

> **Applesauce Cinnamon Crunch Muffins:** *Top the muffins with Cinnamon Sugar Topping (page 225) before baking.*
>
> **Applesauce Crumb Muffins:** *Top the muffins with Crumb Topping (page 226) before baking.*
>
> **Applesauce Granola Muffins:** *Add 1/3 cup granola cereal along with the cinnamon.*
>
> **Applesauce Nut Crunch Muffins:** *Top the muffins with Nut Crunch Topping (page 229) before baking.*
>
> **Applesauce Raisin Muffins:** *Add 1/2 cup golden raisins with the applesauce.*
>
> **Chunky Applesauce Spice Muffins:** *Substitute 1 1/4 cups chunky applesauce for the unsweetened applesauce. Increase the ground cinnamon to 1 teaspoon. Add 1/2 teaspoon ground ginger, 1/4 teaspoon ground cloves, and 1/4 teaspoon ground mace with the cinnamon.*
>
> **Double Apple Applesauce Muffins:** *Add 1/2 cup chopped dried apple with the milk.*
>
> **Heart-Healthy Applesauce Muffins:** *Substitute 1/4 cup plus 2 tablespoons canola oil for the butter. This variation can be used as a base for all the applesauce muffin variations listed here.*
>
> **Sunny Applesauce Muffins:** *Sprinkle 1 teaspoon shelled unsalted sunflower seeds on top of each muffin before baking (about 1/4 cup total).*

Apricot Muffins

Makes 12 muffins

Puréed canned apricots add so much body that these muffins require less fat than some other recipes. Unfortunately, canned apricots lack one thing: a flavor punch. So we've also included dried apricots for a brighter flavor. Dried apricots are sometimes treated with sulfur dioxide so that they will stay colorful on the shelf and glimmer like small jewels in a batter. If you wish to forgo the chemical cosmetics, use the brownish, unsulfured dried apricots available in health food stores and some gourmet markets.

Nonstick spray or paper muffin cups
2$1/4$ cups all-purpose flour
$1/2$ cup sugar
2 teaspoons baking soda
1 teaspoon baking powder
$1/2$ teaspoon ground ginger
$1/2$ teaspoon salt
One 15-ounce can apricot halves in heavy syrup
2 teaspoons lemon juice
$1/4$ teaspoon almond extract
2 large eggs, at room temperature
$1/2$ cup yogurt (regular, low-fat, or nonfat)
$1/3$ cup canola or vegetable oil
1 cup chopped dried apricots

1. Position the rack in the center of the oven and preheat the oven to 400°F. To prepare the muffin tins, spray the indentations and the rims around them with nonstick spray, or line the indentations with paper muffin cups. If using silicon muffin tins, spray as directed, then place them on a baking sheet.

2. Whisk the flour, sugar, baking soda, baking powder, ginger, and salt in a medium bowl until uniform. Set aside.

3. Place the canned apricots with their syrup, lemon juice, and almond extract in a large blender or a food processor fitted with the chopping blade. Pulse 5 or 6 times, or until the mixture blends easily. Scrape down the sides with a rubber spatula, then process or blend for 20 seconds, or until smooth.

4. Whisk the eggs, yogurt, and oil in a large bowl until smooth, then whisk in the prepared apricot purée. With a wooden spoon, stir in the dried apricots and then the flour mixture, just until the apricots are evenly distributed in the batter.

5. Fill the prepared tins three-quarters full. Use additional greased tins or small, ovensafe, greased ramekins for any leftover batter, or reserve the batter for a second baking. Bake for 25 minutes, or until the muffins are lightly browned with rounded tops. A toothpick inserted into the center of one muffin should come out with a crumb or two attached.

6. Set the pan on a wire rack to cool for 10 minutes. Gently tip each muffin to one side to make sure the bottoms are not stuck. If one is, gently rock the muffin back and forth to release it. Remove the muffins from the pan and cool them for 5 minutes more on the rack before serving. If storing or freezing the muffins, cool completely before sealing in an airtight container or freezer-safe plastic bags. The muffins will stay fresh for up to 2 days at room temperature or up to 2 months in the freezer.

> **Apricot Almond Muffins:** *Reduce the chopped dried apricots to 1/2 cup. Add 3/4 cup toasted, slivered almonds with the dried apricots.*
>
> **Apricot Cashew Crunch Muffins:** *Add 1/2 cup chopped, unsalted cashews with the flour. Top the muffins with Cinnamon Sugar Topping (page 225) before baking.*
>
> **Apricot Cinnamon Streusel Muffins:** *Top the muffins with Cinnamon Streusel Topping (page 224) before baking.*
>
> **Apricot Mint Muffins:** *Add 12 large, fresh mint leaves to the food processor or blender with the canned apricots.*
>
> **Apricot Nut Crunch Muffins:** *Top the muffins with Nut Crunch Topping (page 229) before baking.*
>
> **Apricot Oat Crunch Muffins:** *Top the muffins with Oat Crunch Topping (page 230) before baking.*

Banana Muffins

Makes 12 muffins

Using ingredients you probably have on hand, this simple muffin will soon become a breakfast standard in your home. Let your bananas ripen considerably before using them—bananas that turn a little brown and soft on the outside are usually very sweet on the inside. Vinegar in the batter may be a surprise, but adds a subtle contrast, making the muffins taste more like bananas.

Nonstick spray or paper muffin cups
2 cups all-purpose flour
2 teaspoons baking soda
$1/2$ teaspoon salt
$1/2$ teaspoon ground cinnamon
8 tablespoons (1 stick) unsalted butter, at room temperature
1 cup sugar
2 large eggs, at room temperature
3 large, ripe bananas
2 tablespoons milk or half-and-half
1 teaspoon vanilla extract
$1/2$ teaspoon white vinegar

1. Position the rack in the center of the oven and preheat the oven to 400°F. To prepare the muffin tins, spray the indentations and the rims around them with nonstick spray, or line the indentations with paper muffin cups. If using silicon muffin tins, spray as directed, then place them on a baking sheet.

2. Whisk the flour, baking soda, salt, and cinnamon in a medium bowl until uniform. Set aside.

3. In a large bowl, cream the butter and sugar with a wooden spoon until smooth, about 2 minutes. Add the eggs, one at a time, mixing each until well incorporated.

4. Peel the bananas and mash them into the butter mixture using a potato masher. If the bananas are not soft, squeeze them through a potato ricer. Stir in the milk or half-and-half, the vanilla, and vinegar until the mixture is smooth and creamy. Add the prepared flour mixture; stir until moistened.

5. Fill the prepared tins three-quarters full. Use additional greased tins or small, oven-safe, greased ramekins for any leftover batter, or reserve the batter for a second baking. Bake for 18 minutes, or until pale brown with rounded nubbly tops. A toothpick inserted in the center of one muffin should come out with a few moist crumbs attached.

6. Set the pan on a wire rack to cool for 10 minutes. Gently rock each muffin back and forth to release it. Remove the muffins from the pan and cool them for 5 minutes more on the rack before serving. If storing or freezing the muffins, cool them completely before sealing in an airtight container or freezer-safe plastic bags. The muffins will stay fresh for up to 24 hours at room temperature or up to 1 month in the freezer.

> **Banana Chunk Muffins:** *Add 3/4 cup chopped dried bananas with the milk.*
>
> **Banana Coconut Muffins:** *Add 3/4 cup sweetened shredded coconut with the milk.*
>
> **Banana Ginger Muffins:** *Add 1/4 cup finely chopped crystallized ginger with the milk.*
>
> **Banana Nut Crunch Muffins:** *Top the muffins with Nut Crunch Topping (page 229) before baking.*
>
> **Banana Nut Muffins:** *Add 3/4 cup chopped, toasted pecans, walnuts, or hazelnuts with the milk.*
>
> **Banana Pineapple Muffins:** *Add 3/4 cup chopped dried pineapple with the milk.*

Basic Muffins

Makes 12 muffins

If simplicity is your nirvana, look no further for the ultimate muffin. There's nothing fancy here—just an excellent canvas for jam, jelly, or marmalade. The firm crumb also makes these muffins great for sopping up sauces at brunch or dinner. For some more exuberant treats, check out the variations.

Nonstick spray or paper muffin cups
2^1/4 cups all-purpose flour
^{1}/4 cup plus 2 tablespoons sugar
1 tablespoon baking powder
^{1}/2 teaspoon salt
2 large eggs, at room temperature
1^1/4 cups milk (whole, low-fat, or nonfat)
6 tablespoons (^{3}/4 stick) unsalted butter, melted and cooled
1 teaspoon vanilla extract

1. Position the rack in the center of the oven and preheat the oven to 400°F. To prepare the muffin tins, spray the indentations and the rims around them with nonstick spray, or line the indentations with paper muffin cups. If using silicon muffin tins, spray as directed, then place them on a baking sheet.

2. Whisk the flour, sugar, baking powder, and salt in a medium bowl until well combined. Set aside.

3. In a large bowl, lightly whisk the eggs. Whisk in the milk, melted butter, and vanilla. Then stir in the flour mixture with a wooden spoon until moistened.

4. Fill the prepared tins three-quarters full. Use additional greased tins or small, oven-safe, greased ramekins for any leftover batter, or reserve the batter for a second baking. Bake for 18 minutes, or until the muffins are lightly browned with rounded tops. A toothpick inserted into the center of one muffin should come out with a few moist crumbs attached.

5. Set the pan on a wire rack to cool for 10 minutes. Gently rock each muffin back and forth to release it. Remove the muffins from the pan and cool them for 5 minutes more on the rack before serving. If storing or freezing the muffins, cool them

completely before sealing in an airtight container or freezer-safe plastic bags. The muffins will stay fresh for up to 24 hours at room temperature or up to 1 month in the freezer.

Candy Muffins: *Add 3/4 cup of your favorite bite-size chocolate candies with the flour. Possibilities include Reese's Pieces, Raisinettes, or chocolate-covered espresso beans.*

Christmas Morning Muffins: *Add 1 teaspoon rum extract with the milk. Mix 3/4 cup chopped candied fruit into the flour mixture just before adding it to the wet ingredients.*

Crumb Muffins: *Top the muffins with Crumb Topping (page 226) before baking.*

Heart-Healthy Muffins: *Substitute 1/4 cup plus 2 tablespoons canola oil for the butter.*

Nut Crunch Muffins: *Top the muffins with Nut Crunch Topping (page 229) before baking.*

Prune Armagnac Muffins: *Soak 1/2 cup chopped, pitted prunes in 2 tablespoons Armagnac for 1 hour or until the fruit absorbs the liquid. Add the soaked prunes with the milk.*

Rainbow Muffins: *Add 1/2 cup multicolored plain M&M candies with the flour.*

Rum Raisin Muffins: *Soak 1/2 cup raisins in 2 tablespoons dark rum for 1 hour or until the raisins absorb the rum. Add the raisins with the milk.*

Streusel Muffins: *Top the muffins with Cinnamon Streusel Topping (page 224) before baking.*

Thanksgiving Muffins: *Add 1/4 cup dried cranberries and 1/4 cup chopped pecans with the flour. Add 1/2 teaspoon almond extract with the milk.*

White Chocolate Banana Chip Muffins: *Mix in 1/4 cup white chocolate chips and 1/4 cup chopped dried banana with the milk.*

Beer Muffins

Makes 12 muffins

Here's the first of the savory muffins, real treats alongside any meal. Most of the liquid in this batter is beer, which adds both flavor and leavening. We prefer an amber beer, but feel free to experiment with your favorite, so long as it is not a fruit-flavored beer. Start with the beer at room temperature so it doesn't shock the batter and prevent it from rising. The cheese is folded in gently at the end so it can be seen threading the tops of the muffins after they've baked.

Nonstick spray or paper muffin cups
2$^1/_4$ cups all-purpose flour
1$^1/_2$ tablespoons sugar
1 tablespoon baking powder
$^1/_2$ teaspoon salt
$^1/_2$ teaspoon freshly ground black pepper
1 large egg, at room temperature
4 tablespoons ($^1/_2$ stick) unsalted butter, melted and cooled
2 teaspoons Dijon mustard
1$^1/_4$ cups beer, at room temperature
1$^1/_4$ cups shredded sharp Cheddar (about 5 ounces)

1. Position the rack in the center of the oven and preheat the oven to 400°F. To prepare the muffin tins, spray the indentations and the rims around them with nonstick spray, or line the indentations with paper muffin cups. If using silicon muffin tins, spray as directed, then place them on a baking sheet.

2. Whisk the flour, sugar, baking powder, salt, and pepper in a medium bowl until uniform. Set aside.

3. In a large bowl, whisk the egg, melted butter, and mustard until blended. Gently whisk in the beer until the foaming subsides, then add the cheese. Finally, stir in the flour mixture with a wooden spoon until moistened.

4. Fill the prepared tins three-quarters full. Use additional greased tins or small, oven-safe, greased ramekins for any leftover batter, or reserve the batter for a second bak-

ing. Bake for 20 minutes, or until the muffins have lumpy brown tops and a toothpick inserted in the center of one muffin comes out almost clean.

5. Set the pan on a wire rack to cool for 10 minutes. Gently tip each muffin to one side to make sure it's not stuck. If one is, gently rock it back and forth to release it. Remove the muffins from the pan and cool them for 5 minutes more on the rack before serving. If storing or freezing the muffins, cool them completely before sealing in an airtight container or in freezer-safe plastic bags. The muffins will stay fresh for up to 48 hours at room temperature or up to 2 months in the freezer.

Beer Blue Cheese Muffins: *Reduce the Cheddar to 3/4 cup and add 1/2 cup (2 ounces) crumbled blue cheese, such as Gorgonzola or Stilton, with the remaining cheese.*

Beer Caraway Muffins: *Add 1 tablespoon caraway seeds with the flour.*

Beer Celery Seed Muffins: *Add 1 tablespoon celery seeds with the flour.*

Beer Horseradish Muffins: *Add 2 tablespoons bottled prepared horseradish with the mustard.*

Cider Muffins: *Substitute hard cider for the beer.*

Berry Muffins

Makes 12 muffins

We decided to make a set of all-purpose berry muffin recipes—to wit, this recipe, the Low-Fat Berry Muffins (page 112) the Nonfat Berry Muffins (page 138), and the Gluten-Free Berry Muffins (page 94)—rather than different recipes for each kind of berry. Of course, most of us are familiar with the basics—blueberries, raspberries, and blackberries—but there's no reason not to try salmonberries, hulled gooseberries, or fresh currants, if you can find them. The only berry we don't recommend is the venerable but too-wet strawberry—for that, see Strawberry Muffins (page 202). Whichever berry you choose, this batter is hearty enough to stand up to lots of them—it's almost like baking the muffins with jam right inside.

Nonstick spray or paper muffin cups
1³/₄ cups plus 1 tablespoon all-purpose flour
¹/₂ cup oat flour (see A Guide to Some Ingredients, page 11)
¹/₂ cup sugar
1 tablespoon baking powder
¹/₂ teaspoon salt
1 pint berries, hulled if necessary
1 large egg, at room temperature
³/₄ cup buttermilk (regular or low-fat)
8 tablespoons (1 stick) unsalted butter, melted and cooled
1 teaspoon vanilla extract

1. Position the rack in the center of the oven and preheat the oven to 400°F. To prepare the muffin tins, spray the indentations and the rims around them with nonstick spray, or line the indentations with paper muffin cups. If using silicon muffin tins, spray as directed, then place them on a baking sheet.

2. Whisk 1³/₄ cups of the all-purpose flour, the oat flour, sugar, baking powder, and salt in a medium bowl until uniform. In a small bowl, toss the berries with the remaining 1 tablespoon all-purpose flour. Set both bowls aside.

3. In a large bowl, whisk the egg, buttermilk, melted butter, and vanilla until smooth. Use a wooden spoon to stir in the flour mixture just until moistened. Gently fold in the flour-coated berries, incorporating them without breaking them up.

4. Fill the prepared tins three-quarters full. Use additional greased tins or small, oven-safe, greased ramekins for any leftover batter, or reserve the batter for a second baking. Bake for 20 minutes, or until the muffins are browned with cracked but rather flat tops. A toothpick inserted into the center of one muffin should come out with one or two moist crumbs attached, provided the wet berries don't gum up the toothpick as it pierces the muffin.

5. Set the pan on a wire rack to cool for 10 minutes. Gently tip each muffin to one side to make sure it isn't stuck. If so, gently rock it back and forth to release it. Remove the muffins from the pan and cool them upside down on the rack for 5 minutes more before serving. This stops the muffins from collapsing. If storing, cool them completely before sealing in an airtight container. The muffins will stay fresh for up to 2 days at room temperature. Because the berries remain whole, we do not recommend freezing these muffins—they will turn mushy when defrosted.

Berries and Chips Muffins: *Reduce the berries to 1 cup. Toss 2/3 cup semisweet chocolate chips in the flour with the remaining berries.*

Berry Crumb Muffins: *Top the muffins with Crumb Topping (page 226) before baking.*

Berry Crunch Muffins: *Top the muffins with Cinnamon Sugar Topping (page 225) before baking.*

Berry Nut Muffins: *Reduce the berries to 1 cup. Toss 2/3 cup chopped, toasted nuts, such as hazelnuts, pecans, or walnuts, in the flour with the remaining berries.*

Berry Oat Crunch Muffins: *Top the muffins with Oat Crunch Topping (page 230) before baking.*

Berry Streusel Muffins: *Top the muffins with either Cinnamon Streusel Topping (page 224) or Low-Fat Streusel Topping (page 228) before baking.*

Vanilla Glazed Berry Muffins: *Coat the cooled muffins with Vanilla Dip (page 231).*

Black Forest Muffins

Makes 12 muffins

Chocolate and cherries have been immortalized in dozens of sweets, but none so famously as Black Forest cake, a chocolate cake filled with cherries between the layers. For a brighter taste in the muffins inspired by this classic dessert, we use sour cherries, available in cans or jars year-round. Black Forest cake is usually topped with whipped cream, but these muffins could be served with sweetened sour cream or crème fraîche on the side.

Nonstick spray or paper muffin cups
6 tablespoons ($^3/4$ stick) unsalted butter, at room temperature
3 ounces unsweetened chocolate, chopped
3 ounces semisweet chocolate, chopped, or 3 ounces semisweet chocolate chips
2 cups all-purpose flour
2 teaspoons baking powder
1 teaspoon baking soda
1 teaspoon salt
2 eggs, separated, at room temperature
1 cup milk (whole, low-fat, or nonfat)
$^3/4$ cup sugar
$^1/2$ cup sour cream (regular or low–fat, but not nonfat)
1 teaspoon vanilla extract
$^1/4$ teaspoon almond extract
1 cup canned sour cherries, drained and chopped

1. Position the rack in the center of the oven and preheat the oven to 400°F. To prepare the muffin tins, spray the indentations and the rims around them with nonstick spray, or line the indentations with paper muffin cups. If using silicon muffin tins, spray as directed, then place them on a baking sheet.

2. Combine the butter and both kinds of chocolate in the top of a double boiler set over simmering water. If you don't have a double boiler, place the butter and both kinds of chocolate in a heat-safe bowl that fits snugly over a small pan of simmering water. Stir constantly until half the butter and chocolate is melted. Remove the top

of the double boiler or the bowl from the pot, then continue stirring, away from the heat, until the butter and chocolate are completely melted. Cool for 10 minutes.

3. Meanwhile, whisk the flour, baking powder, baking soda, and salt in a medium bowl until well combined. Set aside.

4. In a large bowl, whisk the egg yolks with the milk, sugar, sour cream, vanilla, and almond extract until smooth. Stir in the cooled chocolate mixture and the chopped cherries. Using a wooden spoon, stir in the flour mixture, just until moistened.

5. Fill the prepared tins three-quarters full. Use additional greased tins or small, oven-safe, greased ramekins for any leftover batter, or reserve the batter for a second baking. Bake for 22 minutes, or until the muffins are lightly browned with rounded tops. A toothpick inserted into the center of one muffin should come out clean, provided the cherries don't gum up the tester.

6. Set the pan on a wire rack to cool for 10 minutes. Gently tip each muffin to one side to make sure it isn't stuck. If so, gently rock it back and forth to release it. Remove the muffins from the pan and cool them for 5 minutes more on the rack before serving. If storing or freezing the muffins, cool them completely before sealing in an airtight container or in freezer-safe plastic bags. The muffins will stay fresh for up to 2 days at room temperature or up to 2 months in the freezer.

> **Black Forest Crunch Muffins:** *Top the muffins with Chocolate Crunch Topping (page 222) before baking.*
>
> **Chunky Black Forest Muffins:** *Reduce the sour cherries to 1/2 cup. Mix 1/4 cup dried cherries and 1/2 cup chocolate chips into the flour mixture before adding it to the liquid ingredients.*
>
> **Nutty Black Forest Muffins:** *Mix 1/2 cup chopped sugar-coated cashews or peanuts into the flour mixture before adding it to the liquid ingredients.*

Bran Muffins

Makes 12 muffins

Too often considered hockey pucks or a grim cliché, bran muffins can actually be moist, welcome treats. The secret is not in the amount of bran used, it's in the oil: too much, and the bran turns soggy, the muffins leaden. Reduce the oil, as we've done here, and you'll have light, even healthier muffins every time. For this recipe, use wheat bran, not bran cereal. Look for wheat bran at health food stores or in the baking aisle of most supermarkets.

Nonstick spray or paper muffin cups
$1^2/_3$ cups all-purpose flour
1 cup wheat bran (do not use bran cereal)
2 teaspoons baking soda
1 teaspoon baking powder
$1/_2$ teaspoon salt
$1/_2$ teaspoon ground cinnamon
$1/_4$ teaspoon grated nutmeg
2 large eggs, at room temperature
$1/_2$ cup packed light brown sugar
$1/_2$ cup honey
$1^1/_2$ cups buttermilk (regular or low-fat)
$1/_3$ cup canola or vegetable oil
1 teaspoon vanilla extract
1 cup raisins

1. Position the rack in the center of the oven and preheat the oven to 400°F. To prepare the muffin tins, spray the indentations and the rims around them with nonstick spray, or line the indentations with paper muffin cups. If using silicon muffin tins, spray as directed, then place them on a baking sheet.

2. Whisk the flour, wheat bran, baking soda, baking powder, salt, cinnamon, and nutmeg in a medium bowl until well combined. Set aside.

3. In a large bowl, whisk the eggs, brown sugar, and honey until thick and pale, about 2 minutes. Whisk in the buttermilk, oil, and vanilla, then stir in the raisins. Quickly stir in the flour mixture with a wooden spoon until moistened.

4. Fill the prepared tins three-quarters full. Use additional greased tins or small, oven-safe, greased ramekins for any leftover batter, or reserve the batter for a second baking. Bake for 20 minutes or until the muffins are well browned with high, rounded tops. A toothpick inserted in the center of one muffin should come out clean.

5. Cool the pan on a wire rack for 10 minutes. Gently rock each muffin back and forth to release it. Remove the muffins from the pan and cool them for 5 minutes more on the rack before serving. If storing or freezing the muffins, cool them completely before sealing in an airtight container or in freezer-safe plastic bags. The muffins will stay fresh for up to 2 days at room temperature or up to 2 months in the freezer.

Applesauce Bran Muffins: *Omit the oil. Whisk in 1/3 cup applesauce with the buttermilk.*

Banana Bran Muffins: *Reduce the raisins to 1/2 cup. Add 1 small thinly sliced banana with the remaining raisins.*

Blueberry Bran Muffins: *Substitute dried blueberries for the raisins.*

Cherry Almond Bran Muffins: *Substitute dried cherries for the raisins. Omit the vanilla extract and add 1/2 teaspoon almond extract with the buttermilk.*

Cranberry Bran Muffins: *Substitute dried cranberries for the raisins.*

Orange Bran Muffins: *Reduce the raisins to 1/2 cup. Add one 8-ounce can mandarin orange segments, drained, and 1 teaspoon grated orange zest with the remaining raisins.*

Butterscotch Muffins

Makes 12 muffins

Admittedly, there are many ways to make butterscotch muffins—using melted chips, homemade sauce, or even bottled ice cream topping. All, unfortunately, lead to sticky muffins. We found that the secret is to use butterscotch pudding mix. It makes the muffins sweet and tender, just right for birthday parties, summer picnics, or winter potlucks.

Nonstick spray or paper muffin cups

2 cups all-purpose flour

$^2/_3$ cup sugar

One 3-ounce package butterscotch pudding mix (do not use instant pudding mix)

1 tablespoon baking powder

$^1/_2$ teaspoon salt

1 large egg, at room temperature

1 cup milk (whole, low-fat, or nonfat)

4 tablespoons ($^1/_2$ stick) unsalted butter, melted and cooled

1 teaspoon vanilla extract

1 cup (6 ounces) butterscotch chips

1. Position the rack in the center of the oven and preheat the oven to 400°F. To prepare the muffin tins, spray the indentations and the rims around them with nonstick spray, or line the indentations with paper muffin cups. If using silicon muffin tins, spray as directed, then place them on a baking sheet.

2. Whisk the flour, sugar, pudding mix, baking powder, and salt in a medium bowl until uniform. Set aside.

3. In a large bowl, whisk the egg, milk, melted butter, and vanilla until light and smooth. Stir in the butterscotch chips with a wooden spoon, then quickly stir in the flour mixture until moistened.

4. Fill the prepared tins three-quarters full. Use additional greased tins or small, ovensafe, greased ramekins for any leftover batter, or reserve the batter for a second baking. Bake for 20 minutes, or until the muffins are well browned with smooth

round tops. A toothpick inserted in the center of one muffin should come out with a few moist crumbs attached.

5. Set the pan on a wire rack to cool for 10 minutes. Gently tip each muffin to the side to make sure it isn't stuck. If it is, gently rock it back and forth to release it. Remove the muffins from the pan and cool them for 5 minutes more on the rack before serving. If storing or freezing the muffins, cool them completely before sealing in an airtight container or freezer-safe plastic bags. The muffins will stay fresh for up to 2 days at room temperature or up to 2 months in the freezer.

> **Butterscotch Chocolate Muffins:** *Substitute 3 ounces chocolate pudding mix for the butterscotch pudding mix.*
>
> **Butterscotch Cinnamon Muffins:** *Top the muffins with Cinnamon Sugar Topping (page 225) before baking.*
>
> **Butterscotch Vanilla Almond Muffins:** *Substitute 3 ounces vanilla pudding mix for the butterscotch pudding. Add 1 teaspoon almond extract with the egg. Sprinkle 1 teaspoon sliced almonds on top of each muffin before baking.*
>
> **Butterscotch Walnut Muffins:** *Omit the butterscotch chips. Add 1 cup chopped walnut pieces with the flour.*
>
> **Chocolate Chip Butterscotch Muffins:** *Substitute semisweet chocolate chips for the butterscotch chips.*
>
> **Chocolate Iced Butterscotch Muffins:** *Top the cooled muffins with Chocolate Icing (page 223).*
>
> **Peanut Butter Butterscotch Muffins:** *Substitute peanut butter chips for the butterscotch chips.*

Cappuccino Muffins

Makes 12 muffins

Scalded milk lends that same creamy texture to these muffins as it does to a luxurious cup of cappuccino. Instant espresso powder makes it easy to get that deep, dark coffee taste, but regular or even decaffeinated instant coffee can be used for a lighter take on these decadent muffins. To keep instant espresso powder fresh, store it, tightly covered, in the freezer.

> **Nonstick spray or paper muffin cups**
> **1 cup milk (whole, low-fat, or nonfat)**
> **2 tablespoons instant espresso powder; or 2 tablespoons regular or decaffeinated instant coffee, finely ground in a spice grinder or a coffee grinder**
> **2 cups all-purpose flour**
> **$2/3$ cup sugar**
> **1 tablespoon baking powder**
> **$1/2$ teaspoon salt**
> **1 large egg, at room temperature**
> **8 tablespoons (1 stick) unsalted butter, melted and cooled**
> **2 teaspoons vanilla extract**
> **$1^1/2$ teaspoons ground cinnamon**

1. Position the rack in the center of the oven and preheat the oven to 400°F. To prepare the muffin tins, spray the indentations and the rims around them with nonstick spray, or line the indentations with paper muffin cups. If using silicon muffin tins, spray as directed, then place them on a baking sheet.

2. Scald the milk in a small saucepan over medium-high heat. Once bubbles appear around the pan's rim, remove the milk from the heat and stir in the espresso powder until dissolved. Cool for 5 minutes.

3. Meanwhile, whisk the flour, sugar, baking powder, and salt in a medium bowl until uniform. Set aside.

4. In a large bowl, lightly whisk the egg, then whisk in the melted butter and vanilla until smooth. Whisking all the while, pour in the scalded milk in a thin stream; con-

tinue whisking until completely blended. Using a wooden spoon, quickly stir in the flour mixture until moistened.

5. Fill the prepared tins three-quarters full. Use additional greased tins or small, oven-safe, greased ramekins for any leftover batter, or reserve the batter for a second baking. Sprinkle the cinnamon evenly over the muffins, about 1/8 teaspoon over each muffin. Bake for 18 minutes, or until the tops are slightly cracked and golden brown. A toothpick inserted in the center of one muffin should come out clean.

6. Set the pan on a wire rack to cool for 10 minutes. Gently rock each muffin back and forth to release it. Remove the muffins from the pan and cool them for 5 minutes more on the rack before serving. If storing or freezing the muffins, cool them completely before sealing in an airtight container or in freezer-safe plastic bags. The muffins will stay fresh for up to 24 hours at room temperature or up to 1 month in the freezer.

> **Cappuccino Oreo Muffins:** *Increase the milk by 2 tablespoons. Stir 12 crushed Oreo cookies into the batter just before adding the flour mixture.*
>
> **Chocolate Chip Cappuccino Muffins:** *Allow the steamed milk to cool completely. Stir 3/4 cup semisweet chocolate chips into the batter just before adding the flour mixture.*
>
> **Hazelnut Cappuccino Muffins:** *Reduce the milk to 3/4 cup. Stir 1/4 cup hazelnut-flavored syrup into the remaining milk before scalding. Do not boil or the syrup may crystallize.*
>
> **Walnut Caramel Cappuccino Muffins:** *Reduce the milk to 3/4 cup. Stir 1/4 cup caramel-flavored syrup into the remaining milk before scalding. Also add 2/3 cup chopped walnuts to the batter just before adding the flour mixture.*

Carrot Muffins

Makes 12 muffins

Carrot cake is not exactly healthy, mostly because of the amount of oil needed to keep it moist during the longer baking time a cake requires. With muffins, we can cut down on the oil considerably because they bake so quickly. The result is just as decadent, sure to become a favorite among your friends.

Nonstick spray or paper muffin cups
2 cups all-purpose flour
2 tablespoons granulated sugar
2 teaspoons baking soda
1 teaspoon ground cinnamon
$1/2$ teaspoon salt
$1/4$ teaspoon grated nutmeg
2 large eggs, at room temperature
$1/2$ cup packed light brown sugar
$1/2$ cup canola oil, vegetable oil, or walnut oil
$1/2$ cup buttermilk (regular or low-fat)
$1/2$ cup unsweetened applesauce
1 teaspoon vanilla extract
2 cups shredded carrots (about 4 medium carrots)

1. Position the rack in the center of the oven and preheat the oven to 400°F. To prepare the muffin tins, spray the indentations and the rims around them with nonstick spray, or line the indentations with paper muffin cups. If using silicon muffin tins, spray as directed, then place them on a baking sheet.

2. Whisk the flour, granulated sugar, baking soda, cinnamon, salt, and nutmeg in a medium bowl until uniform. Set aside.

3. In a large bowl, whisk the eggs and brown sugar until thick and pale, about 2 minutes. Whisk in the oil, buttermilk, applesauce, and vanilla until smooth. Using a wooden spoon, stir in the carrots; then quickly stir in the flour mixture until moistened.

4. Fill the prepared tins three-quarters full. Use additional greased tins or small, oven-safe, greased ramekins for any leftover batter, or reserve the batter for a second bak-

ing. Bake for 20 minutes, or until the muffins are well browned. A toothpick inserted in the center of one muffin should come out with a few moist crumbs attached.

5. Set the pan on a wire rack to cool for 10 minutes. Gently tip each muffin to the side to make sure it isn't stuck. If one is, gently rock it back and forth to release it. Remove the muffins from the pan and cool them for 5 minutes more on the rack before serving. If storing or freezing the muffins, cool them completely before sealing in an airtight container or in freezer-safe plastic bags. The muffins will stay fresh for up to 2 days at room temperature or up to 2 months in the freezer.

> **Carrot Coconut Muffins:** *Reduce the shredded carrots to 1 1/2 cups (about 3 medium carrots). Add 1/2 cup unsweetened shredded coconut with the remaining carrots.*
>
> **Carrot Ginger Muffins:** *Add 1/4 cup finely chopped crystallized ginger with the carrots.*
>
> **Carrot Nut Muffins:** *Reduce the shredded carrots to 1 1/2 cups. Add 3/4 cup chopped, toasted nuts, such as almonds, pecans, or walnuts, with the remaining carrots.*
>
> **Carrot Pineapple Muffins:** *Reduce the shredded carrots to 1 1/2 cups. Add 3/4 cup finely chopped dried pineapple with the remaining carrots.*
>
> **Carrot Raisin Muffins:** *Reduce the shredded carrots to 1 1/2 cups. Add 3/4 cup golden raisins with the remaining carrots.*
>
> **Carrot Walnut Cranberry Muffins:** *Use only walnut oil. Reduce the shredded carrots to 1 1/2 cups. Add 3/4 cup dried cranberries with the remaining carrots.*

Cashew Muffins

Makes 12 muffins

Wen toasted, cashews have a soft, sweet flavor, still rich but mellowed considerably. For the best flavor, this recipe uses both cashew butter (found in many supermarkets and in most health food stores) and whole nuts. If you can't find roasted cashews without salt, simply buy raw nuts, spread them on a cookie sheet, and toast them in a 350°F oven for 7 minutes, or until lightly browned and fragrant.

Nonstick spray or paper muffins cups
2 cups all-purpose flour
1 tablespoon baking powder
$^1/_2$ teaspoon salt (see Note)
1 large egg, at room temperature
$^1/_2$ cup packed light brown sugar
1 cup cashew butter
$^1/_4$ cup canola or vegetable oil
1 cup milk (whole, low-fat, or nonfat)
1 teaspoon vanilla extract
$^1/_2$ cup roughly chopped, unsalted, roasted cashews

1. Position the rack in the center of the oven and preheat the oven to 400°F. To prepare the muffin tins, spray the indentations and the rims around them with nonstick spray, or line the indentations with paper muffin cups. If using silicon muffin tins, spray as directed, then place them on a baking sheet. Whisk the flour, baking powder, and salt in a medium bowl until uniform. Set aside.

2. In a large bowl, whisk the egg and brown sugar until thick and pale brown, about 2 minutes. Whisk in the cashew butter and oil; continue whisking until smooth. Then whisk in the milk and vanilla extract. Using a wooden spoon, stir in the chopped cashews, then quickly stir in the flour mixture until moistened.

3. Fill the prepared tins three-quarters full. Use additional greased tins or small, oven-safe, greased ramekins for any leftover batter, or reserve the batter for a second baking. Bake for 20 minutes, or until the muffins have brown, rounded tops. A toothpick inserted in the center of one muffin should come out with a few moist crumbs attached.

4. Set the pan on a wire rack to cool for 10 minutes. Gently rock each muffin back and forth to release it. Remove the muffins from the pan and cool them for 5 minutes more on the rack before serving. If storing or freezing the muffins, cool them completely before sealing in an airtight container or in freezer-safe plastic bags. The muffins will stay fresh for up to 24 hours at room temperature or up to 2 months in the freezer.

Note: *If you're using salted cashew butter, omit the salt in the recipe.*

> **Cashew Cinnamon Crunch Muffins:** *Top the muffins with Cinnamon Streusel Topping (page 224) before baking.*
>
> **Cashew Coconut Muffins:** *Omit the chopped cashews. Add 2/3 cup sweetened shredded coconut with the flour.*
>
> **Cashew Lime Muffins:** *Decrease the milk to 3/4 cup plus 2 tablespoons. Whisk in 2 teaspoons grated lime zest and 2 tablespoons lime juice with the cashew butter. (A Brazilian favorite!)*
>
> **Cashew Raisin Muffins:** *Omit the chopped cashews. Add 2/3 cup raisins with the flour.*

Cheddar Muffins

Makes 12 muffins

Cheddar muffins are a treat—these even more so with a touch of mustard, a few dashes of Tabasco, and a little cornmeal to counter the soft luxury of the cheese. If you can find it, Wisconsin Mammoth Cheddar is a standout in this recipe—it's velvety and aromatic, but firm enough to shred without completely melting into the batter. It's very popular in the Midwest every spring when it's produced.

Nonstick spray or paper muffin cups
2 tablespoons unsalted butter
1 large shallot, finely chopped
2 cups all-purpose flour
1/4 cup yellow or white cornmeal
1/4 cup sugar
1 tablespoon baking powder
1/2 teaspoon salt
1/2 teaspoon freshly ground black pepper
2 cups shredded Cheddar cheese (8 ounces)
2 large eggs, at room temperature
1 cup milk (whole, low-fat, or nonfat)
1/2 cup yogurt (regular, low-fat, or nonfat)
1 tablespoon Dijon mustard
4 dashes Tabasco, or more to taste

1. Position the rack in the center of the oven and preheat the oven to 400°F. To prepare the muffin tins, spray the indentations and the rims around them with nonstick spray, or line the indentations with paper muffin cups. If using silicon muffin tins, spray as directed, then place them on a baking sheet.

2. Melt the butter in a small skillet set over medium heat. Add the shallot and cook for 2 minutes, or until soft and sweet, stirring frequently. Transfer the shallots and any remaining butter in the skillet to a large bowl; cool for 5 minutes.

3. Meanwhile, whisk the flour, cornmeal, sugar, baking powder, salt, and pepper in a medium bowl until uniform. Add the Cheddar and toss until it's coated with the flour. Set aside.

4. Whisk the eggs into the shallots, then whisk in the milk, yogurt, mustard, and Tabasco until smooth. Using a wooden spoon, quickly stir in the flour mixture until moistened.

5. Divide the batter equally among the tins; it will almost fill each indentation to the top. Bake for 25 minutes, or until the tops are slightly cracked and golden brown. A toothpick or cake tester inserted into the center of one muffin should come out with a few moist crumbs attached.

6. Set the pan on a wire rack to cool for 10 minutes. Gently rock each muffin back and forth to release it. Remove the muffins from the pan and cool them for 5 minutes more on the rack before serving. If storing or freezing the muffins, cool them completely before sealing in an airtight container or in freezer-safe plastic bags. The muffins will stay fresh for up to 2 days at room temperature or up to 2 months in the freezer.

> **Cheddar Broccoli Muffins:** *Decrease the cheese to 1 1/2 cups. Add 1 cup chopped frozen broccoli, thawed, with the milk.*
>
> **Cheddar Dill Muffins:** *Add 2 tablespoons chopped fresh dill with the salt and pepper.*
>
> **Cheddar Mushroom Muffins:** *Decrease the cheese to 1 1/2 cups. Add 1/2 cup stemmed and finely chopped shiitake mushrooms or 1/2 cup chopped button mushrooms to the skillet with the shallot. Cook an additional few minutes, or until the mushrooms give off their liquid and it evaporates.*
>
> **Cheddar Pepper Muffins:** *Decrease the cheese to 1 1/2 cups. Add one 4-ounce jar roasted pimientos, drained and roughly chopped, with the milk.*
>
> **Cheddar Sausage Muffins:** *Decrease the cheese to 1 1/2 cups. Add 1 cup crumbled sausage meat to the skillet with the shallot and butter; cook over medium heat until browned, about 5 minutes. Transfer the contents of the skillet to the large bowl.*
>
> **Hungarian Cheddar Muffins:** *Add 2 tablespoons sweet paprika with the salt and pepper. Increase the milk by 1 tablespoon.*

Cheesecake Muffins

Makes 12 muffins

Although too cakey to look like cheesecake, especially with their nubbly tops, these muffins sure taste like the infamous dessert: decadent to the final degree and very creamy, with a layer of sweetened ricotta cheese threading each one.

Nonstick spray or paper muffin cups

2 cups all-purpose flour

2 teaspoons baking soda

1 teaspoon baking powder

$1/2$ teaspoon salt

$1/4$ cup ricotta cheese (whole-milk or low-fat, but not nonfat)

$1/2$ cup plus 2 tablespoons sugar

$1^1/2$ teaspoons vanilla extract

8 ounces cream cheese (regular or low-fat), softened; or 8 ounces Neufchâtel cheese, softened

8 tablespoons (1 stick) unsalted butter, softened

1 large egg, at room temperature

$1/2$ cup buttermilk (regular or low-fat)

2 teaspoons grated lemon zest

1 teaspoon lemon juice

1. Position the rack in the center of the oven and preheat the oven to 375°F. To prepare the muffin tins, spray the indentations and the rims around them with nonstick spray, or line the indentations with paper muffin cups. If using silicon muffin tins, spray as directed, then place them on a baking sheet.

2. Whisk the flour, baking soda, baking powder, and salt in a medium bowl until uniform. Set aside.

3. In a small bowl, mix the ricotta cheese with 2 tablespoons of the sugar and $1/2$ teaspoon of the vanilla until well blended. Set aside as well.

4. In the large bowl, beat the softened cream cheese and the butter with an electric mixer at medium speed about 1 minute, until smooth, scraping down the sides of the bowl as necessary. Continue beating without disturbing until the mixture is light

and pale yellow, about 2 minutes more. Slowly pour in the remaining 1/2 cup sugar, while beating at medium speed for about 3 minutes, or until no sugar can be felt when a little of the mixture is rubbed between your fingertips. Beat in the egg until well incorporated, then beat in the buttermilk, lemon zest, lemon juice, and the remaining 1 teaspoon vanilla.

5. Using a wooden spoon, stir in the prepared flour mixture until moistened.

6. Spoon 2 heaping tablespoons of batter into each muffin cup; gently spread it with the back of the spoon so that it touches the sides of the indentation and is as flat as possible. Mound 1 heaping teaspoon of the ricotta mixture on top of this batter in each muffin cup. Spoon the remaining batter on top of the ricotta filling dividing it evenly between the cups, filling each about three-quarters full.

7. Bake for 25 minutes, or until the tops are bumpy and speckled golden brown. A toothpick or cake tester inserted into the center of one muffin should come out with a few moist crumbs attached, provided you do not press down too far and run into the vein of ricotta cheese.

8. Set the pan on a wire rack to cool for 10 minutes. Gently rock each muffin back and forth to release it. Remove the muffins from the pan and cool them for 5 minutes more on the rack before serving. If storing or freezing the muffins, cool them completely before sealing in an airtight container or in freezer-safe plastic bags. The muffins will stay fresh for up to 2 days at room temperature or up to 2 months in the freezer.

Almond Cheesecake Muffins: *Mix 1/2 cup toasted sliced almonds with the flour mixture. Add 1/2 teaspoon almond extract with the lemon zest and juice.*

Oreo Cheesecake Muffins: *Omit the lemon zest and juice. Stir 1/2 cup crumbled Oreo cookies into the batter before adding the flour mixture.*

Strawberry Cheesecake Muffins: *Reduce the sugar in the batter to 1/2 cup. Omit the sugar completely from the ricotta mixture; instead, stir 1/4 cup strawberry jam into the ricotta cheese with the vanilla. Use 2 teaspoons cheese filling for each muffin.*

White Chocolate Chip Cheesecake Muffins: *Mix 1/2 cup white chocolate chips into the batter before adding the flour mixture.*

Cherry Muffins

Makes 12 muffins

Thank goodness for frozen cherries—they're available all year long and require no pitting. These cherry muffins are so juicy, they almost collapse from the weight of the fruit as they cool. Cool them upside down once you remove them from the muffin tins. A little whole wheat flour adds just the right tooth.

Nonstick spray or paper muffin cups
2 cups all-purpose flour
$1/2$ cup sugar
$1/3$ cup whole wheat flour
2 teaspoons baking soda
1 teaspoon baking powder
$1/2$ teaspoon salt
1 large egg, at room temperature
$1/2$ cup milk (whole, low-fat, or nonfat)
$1/3$ cup sour cream (regular, low-fat, or nonfat)
4 tablespoons ($1/2$ stick) unsalted butter, melted and cooled
$1/2$ teaspoon almond extract
One 10-ounce bag frozen sweet cherries, thawed and roughly chopped

1. Position the rack in the center of the oven and preheat the oven to 400°F. To prepare the muffin tins, spray the indentations and the rims around them with nonstick spray, or line the indentations with paper muffin cups. If using silicon muffin tins, spray as directed, then place them on a baking sheet.

2. Whisk the all-purpose flour, sugar, whole wheat flour, baking soda, baking powder, and salt in a medium bowl until uniform. Set aside.

3. In a large bowl, whisk the egg until lightly beaten, then whisk in the milk, sour cream, melted butter, and almond extract until smooth. Using a wooden spoon, stir in the cherries, then quickly stir in the flour mixture until moistened.

4. Fill the prepared tins three-quarters full. Use additional greased tins or small, oven-safe, greased ramekins for any leftover batter, or reserve the batter for a second baking. Bake for 22 minutes, or until the tops are browned and somewhat flat like

shiitake mushroom caps. A toothpick inserted in the center of one muffin should come out almost clean, provided the cherries don't gum up the tester.

5. Set the pan on a wire rack to cool for 10 minutes. Gently tip each muffin to the side to make sure it isn't stuck. If it is, gently rock it back and forth to release it. Remove the muffins from the pan and cool them upside down for 5 minutes more on the rack before serving. This stops the muffins from collapsing. If storing or freezing the muffins, cool them completely before sealing in an airtight container or in freezer-safe plastic bags. The muffins will stay fresh for up to 2 days at room temperature or up to 2 months in the freezer.

> **Cherry Chocolate Chip Muffins:** *Add 1/2 cup semisweet chocolate chips with the cherries.*
>
> **Cherry Chocolate Crunch Muffins:** *Top the muffins with Chocolate Crunch Topping (page 222) before baking.*
>
> **Cherry Lime Ricky Muffins:** *Reduce the milk to 3/4 cup. Add 1/4 cup limeade concentrate with the remaining milk.*
>
> **Cherry Nut Crunch Muffins:** *Top the muffins with Nut Crunch Topping (page 229) before baking.*
>
> **Cherry Vanilla Glazed Muffins:** *Coat the cooled muffins with Vanilla Dip (page 231).*
>
> **Chocolate Iced Cherry Muffins:** *Top the cooled muffins with Chocolate Icing (page 223).*
>
> **Extra Almond Cherry Muffins:** *Omit the whole wheat flour. Add 1/3 cup ground almonds with the flour.*

Chestnut Muffins

Makes 12 muffins

Since fresh chestnuts can be dry, sweetened canned chestnut purée is a good alternative for baking. It has glucose and other sugars which preserve most of the moisture and ensure that nutty, slightly coarse texture so favored among chestnut lovers. You can find sweetened chestnut purée in the baking aisle of most supermarkets. To make these muffins complete, try them with a pat of butter and a drizzle of chestnut honey (see Source Guide, page 237).

Nonstick spray or paper muffin cups
2 cups all-purpose flour
$^1/_2$ cup whole wheat flour
1 tablespoon baking powder
$^1/_2$ teaspoon salt
1 large egg, at room temperature
$^1/_4$ cup packed light brown sugar
One $8^3/_4$-ounce can sweetened chestnut purée
6 tablespoons ($^3/_4$ stick) unsalted butter, melted and cooled
2 teaspoons vanilla extract
1 cup milk (whole or low-fat, but not nonfat)

1. Position the rack in the center of the oven and preheat the oven to 400°F. To prepare the muffin tins, spray the indentations and the rims around them with nonstick spray, or line the indentations with paper muffin cups. If using silicon muffin tins, spray as directed, then place them on a baking sheet.

2. Whisk the all-purpose flour, whole wheat flour, baking powder, and salt in a medium bowl until uniform. Set aside.

3. In a large bowl, whisk the egg until lightly beaten, then whisk in the brown sugar. Continue whisking until the mixture is smooth, thick, and pale brown, about 3 minutes. Whisk in the chestnut purée, melted butter, and vanilla until smooth.

4. Whisking the egg-sugar mixture all the while, pour in the milk in a thin, steady stream. Once the mixture is smooth, use a wooden spoon to stir in the flour mixture until moistened.

5. Fill the prepared tins three-quarters full. Use additional greased tins or small, oven-safe, greased ramekins for any leftover batter, or reserve the batter for a second baking. Bake for 20 minutes, or until the muffins have lightly browned, rounded tops. A toothpick inserted in the center of one muffin should come out clean.

6. Set the pan on a wire rack to cool for 10 minutes. Gently rock each muffin back and forth to release it. Remove the muffins from the pan and cool them for 5 minutes more on the rack before serving. If storing or freezing the muffins, cool them completely before sealing in an airtight container or in freezer-safe plastic bags. The muffins will stay fresh for up to 24 hours at room temperature or up to 2 months in the freezer.

Chestnut Cherry Muffins: *Stir 1/2 cup chopped glacéed cherries into the batter before adding the flour mixture.*

Chestnut Cinnamon Crunch Muffins: *Top the muffins with Cinnamon Sugar Topping (page 225) before baking.*

Chestnut Honey Muffins: *Omit the brown sugar. Whisk in 1/4 cup dark honey, such as chestnut, pine, or buckwheat, with the egg.*

Chestnut Orange Muffins: *Add 1/2 cup chopped candied orange rind with the chestnut purée.*

Vanilla Glazed Chestnut Muffins: *Coat the cooled muffins with Vanilla Dip (page 231).*

Chocolate Angel Food Muffins

Makes 12 muffins

Denser than Angel Food Muffins (page 20) but lighter than Cocoa Muffins (page 64), these are perfect for chocolate lovers who want a treat that won't blow their diets. The taste is purely chocolate, especially if you use a high quality cocoa powder. But the final product is light as air, only slightly heavier than chocolate meringue cookies.

Nonstick spray for the muffin tins
1/2 cup all-purpose flour, plus additional for the muffin tins
1 cup plus 3 tablespoons sugar
1/2 cup cocoa powder, sifted
12 large egg whites, at room temperature
1/2 teaspoon salt
1 teaspoon cream of tartar
2 teaspoons vanilla extract

1. Position the rack in the center of the oven and preheat the oven to 375°F. To prepare the muffin tins, spray the indentations and the rim around them with nonstick spray. Sprinkle a pinch of flour into each of the indentations and shake the tin around, rapping your hands on the bottom and sides to coat the interior surface of the muffin cups with flour. Shake out any excess flour by rapping the tin against the side of the sink. If you're using silicon muffin tins, forgo dusting them with flour—simply spray the tins and place the tins on a baking sheet.

2. Whisk the flour, 1/2 cup of the sugar, and the cocoa powder in a medium bowl until uniform. Set aside.

3. Place the egg whites and salt in a large bowl. Beat with an electric mixer at medium speed until frothy. Add the cream of tartar and beat at high speed until soft peaks form. With the mixer running, add the remaining 1/2 cup plus 3 tablespoons sugar in a slow stream. Once the sugar has been added, beat in the vanilla. Continue beating for 3 minutes, or until the mixture is stiff and shiny and no sugar granules can be felt when a bit of the egg whites is rubbed between your fingertips.

4. Fold in one third of the flour mixture with a rubber spatula. Using long, even arcs, incorporate the flour evenly into the egg white mixture. Fold in half of the remaining flour mixture using the same technique. Once incorporated, fold in the remainder of the flour mixture very gently, taking care not to mash down the egg whites. The final addition will not dissolve, but the flour should be evenly distributed.

5. Divide the batter evenly among the muffin tins; fill them high, since the muffins will not rise as they bake. Bake for 30 minutes, or until the tops are dry and lightly browned.

6. Transfer the tins to a cooling rack and cool for 45 minutes before attempting to remove the muffins. Gently rock each muffin back and forth to release it from the tin. Store these muffins in an airtight container at room temperature for up to 24 hours or in the freezer for up to 3 months.

> **Chocolate Cinnamon Angel Food Muffins:** *Whisk 1 teaspoon ground cinnamon into the flour mixture.*
>
> **Chocolate Orange Angel Food Muffins:** *Add 1 teaspoon orange extract or 1/4 teaspoon orange oil with the vanilla.*
>
> **Chocolate Rum Angel Food Muffins:** *Add 1 teaspoon rum extract with the vanilla.*
>
> **Mexican Chocolate Angel Food Muffins:** *Substitute 1/2 teaspoon almond extract for the vanilla. Whisk 1 teaspoon ground cinnamon into the flour mixture. Stir 1/2 cup cocoa nibs into the batter with the last addition of the flour mixture.*

Chocolate Chip Muffins

Makes 12 muffins

Chocolate chip muffins may inspire turf wars, but these might suit all sides. They're a little sweeter than some of the other muffins in this book so that the taste of the chocolate really comes through. The egg whites are beaten separately, a seemingly fussy step that actually lightens a batter laced so heavily with chocolate chips. And sour cream adds a slight tang that enhances both the chocolate and vanilla flavors.

Nonstick spray or paper muffin cups
2^1/4 cups all-purpose flour
^{1}/3 cup granulated sugar
2 teaspoons baking powder
^{1}/2 teaspoon salt
1 cup semisweet chocolate chips
2 large eggs, separated, at room temperature
^{1}/2 cup sour cream (regular, low-fat, or nonfat)
^{1}/2 cup packed light brown sugar
6 tablespoons (^{3}/4 stick) unsalted butter, melted and cooled
1 teaspoon vanilla extract
1 cup milk (whole, low-fat, or nonfat)

1. Position the rack in the center of the oven and preheat the oven to 400°F. To prepare the muffin tins, spray the indentations and the rims around them with nonstick spray, or line the indentations with paper muffin cups. If using silicon muffin tins, spray as directed, then place them on a baking sheet.

2. Whisk the flour, granulated sugar, baking powder, and salt in a medium bowl until uniform. Stir in the chocolate chips until well coated with flour. Set aside.

3. In a second medium bowl, beat the egg whites with an electric mixer at high speed for 2 minutes, or until soft, airy peaks form. Set aside.

4. In a large bowl, whisk the egg yolks with the sour cream, brown sugar, melted butter, and vanilla for 2 minutes, or until the mixture is light, smooth, and pale brown. Whisk in the milk until uniformly blended, about 30 seconds.

5. Using a wooden spoon, stir in the flour mixture until moistened, then gently fold in the egg whites just until no white streaks are visible.

6. Fill the prepared tins three-quarters full. Use additional greased tins or small, oven-safe, greased ramekins for any leftover batter, or reserve the batter for a second baking. Bake for 23 minutes, or until the tops are slightly cracked and lightly browned.

7. Set the pan on a wire rack to cool for 10 minutes. Gently rock each muffin back and forth to release it. Remove the muffins from the pan and cool them for 5 minutes more on the rack before serving. If storing or freezing the muffins, cool them completely before sealing in an airtight container or in freezer-safe plastic bags. The muffins will stay fresh for up to two days at room temperature or up to 2 months in the freezer.

> **Carob Chip Muffins:** *Substitute 1 cup carob chips for the semisweet chocolate chips.*
>
> **Chocolate Chip Chocolate Crunch Muffins:** *Top each muffin with Chocolate Crunch Topping (page 222) before baking.*
>
> **Milk Chocolate Chip Muffins:** *Substitute 1 cup milk chocolate chips for the semisweet chips.*
>
> **Mint Chocolate Chip Muffins:** *Substitute 1 teaspoon mint extract for the vanilla extract. Substitute 1 cup shaved dark chocolate or dark chocolate mini chips for the semisweet chips.*

Chocolate Chocolate Chip Muffins

Makes 12 muffins

Although these muffins are indulgent to the nth degree, they're not quite sweet enough to cross the line into cupcakes—although they'd be terrific as a dessert any night of the week. To go over the top, serve these with Nutella, a hazelnut chocolate spread, available in most supermarkets.

Nonstick spray or paper muffin cups
2 cups all-purpose flour
$1/2$ cup granulated sugar
$1/3$ cup cocoa powder, sifted
2 teaspoons baking soda
1 teaspoon baking powder
$1/2$ teaspoon salt
1 cup semisweet chocolate chips
2 large eggs, at room temperature
$1/4$ cup packed dark brown sugar
$1^1/2$ cups buttermilk (regular or low-fat)
8 tablespoons (1 stick) unsalted butter, melted and cooled
1 teaspoon vanilla extract

1. Position the rack in the center of the oven and preheat the oven to 400°F. To prepare the muffin tins, spray the indentations and the rims around them with nonstick spray, or line the indentations with paper muffin cups. If using silicon muffin tins, spray as directed, then place them on a baking sheet.

2. Whisk the flour, granulated sugar, cocoa powder, baking soda, baking powder, and salt in a medium bowl until uniform. Stir in the chocolate chips until well coated. Set aside.

3. In a large bowl, whisk the eggs and brown sugar until thick and pale brown, about 2 minutes. Pour in the buttermilk, melted butter, and vanilla; whisk until smooth. Using a wooden spoon, stir in the flour mixture until moistened.

4. Fill the prepared tins three-quarters full. Use additional greased tins or small, oven-safe, greased ramekins for any leftover batter, or reserve the batter for a second bak-

ing. Bake for 20 minutes, or until the muffins are lightly browned with rounded tops. A toothpick inserted into the center of one muffin should come out clean, unless you hit a chocolate chip.

5. Set the pan on a wire rack to cool for 10 minutes. Gently tip each muffin to one side to make sure it isn't stuck. If one is, gently rock it back and forth to release it. Remove the muffins from the pan and cool them for 5 minutes more on the rack before serving. If storing or freezing the muffins, cool them completely before sealing in an airtight container or in freezer-safe plastic bags. The muffins will stay fresh for up to 2 days at room temperature or up to 2 months in the freezer.

> **Black and White Chocolate Chocolate Chip Muffins:** *Sprinkle 6 white chocolate chips onto the top of each muffin before baking (about 1/4 cup white chocolate chips in total).*
>
> **Cherry Chocolate Chocolate Chip Muffins:** *Reduce chocolate chips to 1/2 cup. Stir 1/2 cup dried cherries into the flour mixture with the remaining chocolate chips.*
>
> **Chocolate Peanut Butter Chip Muffins:** *Substitute peanut butter chips for the semisweet chocolate chips.*
>
> **Mint Chocolate Chocolate Chip Muffins:** *Add 2 teaspoons mint extract to the liquid ingredients with the buttermilk.*
>
> **Rainbow Chocolate Chocolate Chip Muffins:** *Sprinkle 8 M&M baking bits candies on the top of each muffin before baking (about 1/4 cup M&M baking bits in total).*

Chocolate Malt Muffins

Makes 12 muffins

Malt is made from sprouted barley that has been dried and ground to a fine powder. In muffins, it takes on an entirely new character when baked with chocolate: softer, yet somehow more complex, with a slight herbal taste. These muffins cry out for sweetened sour cream or crème fraîche.

Nonstick spray or paper muffin cups
1 cup milk (whole, low-fat, or nonfat)
$^3/_4$ cup malted milk powder
2 cups all-purpose flour
2 teaspoons baking soda
$^1/_2$ teaspoon baking powder
$^1/_2$ teaspoon salt
3 ounces unsweetened chocolate, chopped
6 tablespoons ($^3/_4$ stick) unsalted butter, at room temperature
2 large eggs, at room temperature
1 cup sugar
1 teaspoon vanilla extract

1. Position the rack in the center of the oven and preheat the oven to 400°F. To prepare the muffin tins, spray the indentations and the rims around them with nonstick spray, or line the indentations with paper muffin cups. If using silicon muffin tins, spray as directed, then place them on a baking sheet.

2. Whisk the milk and malted milk powder in a small bowl until the malt dissolves. Let stand at room temperature for 15 minutes.

3. Meanwhile, whisk the flour, baking soda, baking powder, and salt in a medium bowl until uniform. Set aside.

4. Place the chocolate and butter in the top of a double boiler set over simmering water. If you don't have a double boiler, place the chocolate and butter in a heat-safe bowl that fits snugly over a small pot of simmering water. Stir constantly until half the butter and chocolate is melted. Remove the top of the double boiler or the bowl

from the pot; then continue stirring, away from the heat, until the butter and chocolate are completely smooth. Cool for 5 minutes.

5. In a large bowl, whisk the eggs until lightly beaten, then pour in the sugar and continue whisking until the mixture is thick and pale yellow, about 3 minutes. Stir in the vanilla, then the prepared malt mixture. Pour in the cooled chocolate mixture in a slow, steady stream, whisking all the while. Finally, use a wooden spoon to stir in the flour mixture, just until moistened.

6. Fill the prepared tins three-quarters full. Use additional greased tins or small, oven-safe, greased ramekins for any leftover batter, or reserve the batter for a second baking. Bake for 20 minutes, or until the muffins have cracked, rounded tops, and a toothpick inserted in the center of one muffin comes out clean.

7. Set the pan on a wire rack to cool for 10 minutes. Gently rock each muffin back and forth to release it. Remove the muffins from the pan and cool for 5 minutes more on the rack before serving. If storing or freezing the muffins, cool them completely before sealing in an airtight container or in freezer-safe plastic bags. The muffins will stay fresh for up to 24 hours at room temperature or up to 2 months in the freezer.

Chocolate Almond Malt Muffins: *Add 1 teaspoon almond extract with the vanilla. Add 1/2 cup sliced almonds with the melted chocolate mixture.*

Chocolate Banana Malt Muffins: *Add 3/4 cup chopped dried banana with the melted chocolate mixture.*

Chocolate Cherry Malt Muffins: *Add 3/4 cup chopped dried cherries with the melted chocolate mixture.*

Chocolate Chip Chocolate Malt Muffins: *Add 1 cup semisweet chocolate chips with the flour.*

Chocolate Malt Crunch Muffins: *Top the muffins with Chocolate Crunch Topping (page 222) before baking.*

Cocoa Muffins

Makes 12 muffins

These dark-as-night, dense, chewy muffins use the intense flavor of cocoa powder for a chocolate lover's fix. They're just right with a pat of butter and a glass of milk or a cup of coffee.

Nonstick spray or paper muffin cups
2 cups all-purpose flour
$^3/_4$ cup sugar
$^1/_2$ cup cocoa powder, sifted
1 tablespoon baking powder
$^1/_2$ teaspoon salt
2 eggs, at room temperature
$1^1/_4$ cups milk (whole or low-fat, but not nonfat)
$^1/_3$ cup canola or vegetable oil
2 teaspoons vanilla extract

1. Position the rack in the center of the oven and preheat the oven to 400°F. To prepare the muffin tins, spray the indentations and the rims around them with nonstick spray, or line the indentations with paper muffin cups. If using silicon muffin tins, spray as directed, then place them on a baking sheet.

2. Whisk the flour, sugar, cocoa powder, baking powder, and salt in a medium bowl until uniform. Set aside.

3. In a large bowl, whisk the eggs until lightly beaten, then whisk in the milk, oil, and vanilla until smooth. Stir in the prepared flour mixture with a wooden spoon until moistened.

4. Fill the prepared tins three-quarters full. Use additional greased tins or small, oven-safe, greased ramekins for any leftover batter, or reserve the batter for a second baking. Bake for 23 minutes or until the muffins have firm, rounded tops, and a toothpick inserted into the center of one muffin comes out with a few moist crumbs attached.

5. Set the pan on a wire rack to cool for 10 minutes. Gently rock each muffin back and forth to release it. Remove the muffins from the pan and cool for 5 minutes more

on the rack before serving. If storing or freezing the muffins, cool them completely before sealing in an airtight container or in freezer-safe plastic bags. The muffins will stay fresh for up to 24 hours at room temperature or up to 2 months in the freezer.

Chocolate Iced Cocoa Muffins: *Top the cooled muffins with Chocolate Icing (page 223).*

Cocoa Almond Crunch Muffins: *Reduce the vanilla to 1 teaspoon. Add 1 teaspoon almond extract with the vanilla. Top the muffins with Nut Crunch Topping (page 229) before baking.*

Cocoa Cherry Crunch Muffins: *Add 1/2 cup dried cherries with the flour. Top the muffins with Chocolate Crunch Topping (page 222) before baking.*

Cocoa Cranberry Walnut Muffins: *Add 1/2 cup chopped walnuts and 1/2 cup dried cranberries with the flour.*

Cocoa Marshmallow Muffins: *Add 3/4 cup miniature marshmallows to the batter before stirring in the dry ingredients.*

Cocoa Nib Muffins: *Add 3/4 cup chopped cocoa nibs with the flour.*

Coconut Muffins

Makes 12 muffins

Unsweetened shredded coconut and coconut milk give these muffins a velvety texture and an exotic flavor. Both add the true flavor of coconut without masking it behind sugar. For a change of pace, bring these muffins to your next beach picnic, or serve them with tropical drinks in the dead of winter.

Nonstick spray or paper muffin cups

1^1/2 cups unsweetened coconut flakes (see A Guide to Some Ingredients, page 11)

1 tablespoon plus 1 teaspoon packed dark brown sugar

10 tablespoons (1^1/4 sticks) unsalted butter, melted and cooled

2 cups all-purpose flour

^{2}/3 cup granulated sugar

2 teaspoons baking powder

^{1}/2 teaspoon baking soda

^{1}/2 teaspoon salt

2 large eggs, at room temperature

One 5^1/2-ounce can (^{1}/2 cup plus 2 tablespoons) unsweetened coconut milk (see A Guide to Some Ingredients, page 11)

^{1}/4 cup milk (whole, low-fat, or nonfat)

1 teaspoon grated lemon zest

1. Position the rack in the center of the oven and preheat the oven to 400°F. To prepare the muffin tins, spray the indentations and the rims around them with nonstick spray, or line the indentations with paper muffin cups. If using silicon muffin tins, spray as directed, then place them on a baking sheet.

2. Place the 1/4 cup of the coconut flakes and the brown sugar in a food processor fitted with the chopping blade; pulse until coarsely ground. Transfer the mixture to a small bowl and stir in 4 tablespoons (1/4 cup) of the melted butter. Set aside.

3. Whisk the flour, granulated sugar, baking powder, baking soda, and salt in a medium bowl until well combined. Stir in the remaining 1^1/4 cups coconut flakes until thoroughly coated. Set aside as well.

4. In a large bowl, whisk the eggs until lightly beaten, then whisk in the coconut milk, milk, lemon zest, and the remaining melted butter. Stir in the prepared flour mixture with a wooden spoon until moistened.

5. Fill the prepared tins three-quarters full. Use additional greased tins or small, oven-safe, greased ramekins for any leftover batter, or reserve the batter for a second baking. Sprinkle about 1 1/2 teaspoons of the reserved coconut and brown sugar mixture on top of each muffin. Bake for 25 minutes, or until the muffins are lightly golden brown with rounded tops. A toothpick inserted into the center of one muffin should come out with a crumb or two attached.

6. Set the pan on a wire rack to cool for 10 minutes. Gently tip each muffin to the side to make sure it isn't stuck. If one is, gently rock it back and forth to release it. Remove the muffins from the pan and cool for 5 minutes more on the rack before serving. If storing or freezing the muffins, cool them completely before sealing in an airtight container or in freezer-safe plastic bags. The muffins will stay fresh for up to 2 days at room temperature or up to 3 months in the freezer.

> **Chocolate Coconut Muffins:** *Stir 1/2 cup semisweet chocolate chips into the flour mixture with the coconut flakes.*
>
> **Coconut Banana Muffins:** *Add 1/2 cup chopped dried banana into the flour mixture with the coconut flakes.*
>
> **Coconut Rum Muffins:** *Stir 1 teaspoon rum extract with the lemon zest.*
>
> **Sweet Tooth Coconut Muffins:** *Reduce the unsweetened coconut flakes to 1/4 cup. Stir 1 1/4 cups sweetened shredded coconut into the egg mixture before adding the dry ingredients.*

Coffeecake Muffins

Makes 12 muffins

These would make a great centerpiece for Sunday brunch. The light, delicate muffin surrounds a buttery cinnamon filling, much as in a traditional coffeecake, but with the characteristic muffin texture. If you're selling your house, bake up a batch of these to leverage a higher price. Toast the walnut pieces in a dry skillet set over low heat for about 4 minutes, or until very fragrant; then grind them in a spice grinder or a mini food processor.

Nonstick spray or paper muffin cups
$1/2$ cup toasted walnut pieces, coarsely ground (see Note)
8 tablespoons (1 stick) unsalted butter, melted and cooled
2 tablespoons packed light brown sugar
1 tablespoon maple syrup
$1/2$ teaspoon ground cinnamon
$3/4$ teaspoon salt
2 large eggs, separated, at room temperature
2 cups all-purpose flour
$2/3$ cup granulated sugar
1 tablespoon baking powder
1 cup buttermilk (regular, low-fat, or nonfat)
1 teaspoon vanilla extract

1. Position the rack in the center of the oven and preheat the oven to 400°F. To prepare the muffin tins, spray the indentations and the rims around them with nonstick spray, or line the indentations with paper muffin cups. If using silicon muffin tins, spray as directed, then place them on a baking sheet.

2. To make the filling for the muffins, stir the ground walnuts, 3 tablespoons melted butter, brown sugar, maple syrup, cinnamon, and 1/4 teaspoon of the salt in a small bowl until well blended. Set aside.

3. Beat the egg whites in a second medium bowl with an electric mixer at high speed until stiff but moist peaks form, about 2 minutes. Set aside.

4. In a small bowl, whisk the flour, granulated sugar, baking powder, and the remaining 1/2 teaspoon of salt until uniform. Set aside as well.

5. In a large bowl, whisk the egg yolks, buttermilk, the remaining melted butter, and vanilla until smooth. Stir in the flour mixture with a rubber spatula until moistened. Then gently fold in the beaten whites just until no streaks of white are visible.

6. Fill the prepared muffin tins halfway with batter, smoothing it out to meet the sides of the indentations. Top each with 1 tablespoon of the cinnamon and walnut mixture. Divide the remaining batter equally among the tins, filling them three-quarters full. Bake for 20 minutes, or until the muffins are well browned and a toothpick inserted in the center of one muffin comes out with a few moist crumbs attached.

7. Set the pan on a wire rack to cool for 10 minutes. Gently rock each muffin back and forth to release it. Remove the muffins from the pan and cool for 5 minutes more on the rack before serving. If storing or freezing the muffins, cool them completely before sealing in an airtight container or in freezer-safe plastic bags. The muffins will stay fresh for up to 24 hours at room temperature or up to 2 months in the freezer.

Note: *Walnut pieces can be toasted on a baking sheet in a 350°F oven for about 5 minutes, stirring occasionally, until lightly browned and aromatic.*

> **Chocolate Chip Coffeecake Muffins:** *Add 1/2 cup semisweet chocolate chips to the batter before stirring in the flour mixture.*
>
> **Coffeecake Nut Crunch Muffins:** *Top the muffins with Nut Crunch Topping (page 229) before baking.*
>
> **Fig Coffeecake Muffins:** *Add 1/2 cup chopped dried figs to the batter before stirring in the flour mixture.*
>
> **Vanilla Glazed Coffeecake Muffins:** *Coat the cooled muffins with Vanilla Dip (page 231).*

Cola Muffins

Makes 12 muffins

These are not for the faint of . . . well, sweet tooth. In the South, cola cakes, chock full of chocolate and mini marshmallows, are common at any potluck, from family reunions to church picnics. The cola's carbonation even leavens the batter. These muffins pay homage to that old-time cake recipe; they're great for after school treats or a snack during a car trip.

> **Nonstick spray or paper muffin cups**
> 1 cup (6 ounces) semisweet chocolate chips, or 6 ounces semisweet chocolate, chopped
> 6 tablespoons ($^3/4$ stick) unsalted butter, at room temperature
> $2^1/4$ cups all-purpose flour
> $^1/2$ cup sugar
> 1 tablespoon baking powder
> $^1/2$ teaspoon salt
> 1 large egg, at room temperature
> $^1/2$ cup milk (whole, low-fat, or nonfat)
> 2 teaspoons vanilla extract
> 1 cup cola, at room temperature
> $^2/3$ cup mini marshmallows

1. Position the rack in the center of the oven and preheat the oven to 400°F. To prepare the muffin tins, spray the indentations and the rims around them with nonstick spray, or line the indentations with paper muffin cups. If using silicon muffin tins, spray as directed, then place them on a baking sheet.

2. Place the chocolate and butter in the top of a double boiler set over simmering water. If you don't have a double boiler, place the chocolate and butter in a heat-safe bowl that fits snugly over a small pot of simmering water. Stir constantly until half the chocolate and butter is melted. Remove the top of the double boiler or the bowl from the pot; then continue stirring, away from the heat, until the butter and chocolate are completely smooth. Cool for 10 minutes.

3. Meanwhile, whisk the flour, sugar, baking powder, and salt in a medium bowl until uniform. Set aside.

4. In a large bowl, whisk the egg, milk, and vanilla until smooth. Whisking all the while, slowly pour in the cooled chocolate mixture; continue whisking until well blended.

5. Use a wooden spoon to stir in half the flour mixture. Gently stir in the cola. When the foaming subsides, stir in the remaining flour mixture and the mini marshmallows just until the flour is moistened.

6. Fill the prepared tins three-quarters full. Use additional greased tins or small, oven-safe, greased ramekins for any leftover batter, or reserve the batter for a second baking. Bake for 20 minutes, or until the muffins have rounded cracked tops and a toothpick inserted in the center of one muffin comes out with a few moist crumbs attached.

7. Set the pan on a wire rack to cool for 10 minutes. Gently rock each muffin back and forth to release it. Remove the muffins from the pan and cool for 5 minutes more on the rack before serving. If storing or freezing the muffins, cool them completely before sealing in an airtight container or in freezer-safe plastic bags. The muffins will stay fresh for up to 24 hours at room temperature or up to 1 month in the freezer.

Black Cherry Cola Muffins: *Substitute black cherry soda for the cola. Add 1/2 cup pitted fresh black cherries or frozen black cherries, thawed, with the marshmallows.*

Dr Pepper Muffins: *Substitute Dr Pepper for the cola.*

Pecan Cola Muffins: *Add 1/2 cup chopped toasted pecan pieces with the flour.*

Root Beer Float Muffins: *Substitute root beer for the cola. When cooled, coat the muffins with Vanilla Dip (page 231).*

Corn Muffins

Makes 12 muffins

We have definite requirements for corn muffins: they should be decadent, but not too sweet. There's nothing worse than cloying cornbread. So these muffins are our idea of heaven—with sour cream, buttermilk, and butter.

Nonstick spray or paper muffin cups
1¹/2 cups yellow cornmeal
1 cup all-purpose flour
3 tablespoons sugar
2¹/2 teaspoons baking soda
1/2 teaspoon baking powder
1/2 teaspoon salt
2 large eggs, at room temperature
1 cup buttermilk (regular or low-fat)
2/3 cup sour cream (regular or low-fat, but not nonfat)
4 tablespoons (1/2 stick) unsalted butter, melted and cooled

1. Position the rack in the center of the oven and preheat the oven to 375°F. To prepare the muffin tins, spray the indentations and the rims around them with nonstick spray, or line the indentations with paper muffin cups. If using silicon muffin tins, spray as directed, then place them on a baking sheet.

2. Whisk the cornmeal, flour, sugar, baking soda, baking powder, and salt in a medium bowl until uniform. Set aside.

3. In a large bowl, whisk the eggs until lightly beaten, then whisk in the buttermilk, sour cream, and melted butter until smooth. Stir in the cornmeal mixture with a wooden spoon until incorporated.

4. Fill the prepared tins three-quarters full. Use additional greased tins or small, oven-safe, greased ramekins for any leftover batter, or reserve the batter for a second baking. Bake for 22 minutes, or until the muffins have bumpy rounded tops and a toothpick inserted in the center of one muffin comes out clean.

5. Set the pan on a wire rack to cool for 10 minutes. Gently rock each muffin back and forth to release it. Remove the muffins from the pan and cool for 5 minutes more

on the rack before serving. If storing or freezing the muffins, cool them completely before sealing in an airtight container or in freezer-safe plastic bags. The muffins will stay fresh for up to 24 hours at room temperature or up to 1 month in the freezer.

Blue Cheese Corn Muffins: *Stir in 1/2 cup crumbled blue cheese, such as Gorgonzola or Danish blue, before adding the flour mixture.*

Corn Dog Muffins: *Toss 2 hot dogs, sliced into 1/2-inch rings, with the flour mixture before adding it to the batter.*

Ham and Cheese Corn Muffins: *Add 1/2 cup chopped smoked ham and 1/4 cup diced Swiss cheese with the buttermilk.*

Olive Corn Muffins: *Add 1/2 cup sliced pitted black olives with the buttermilk.*

Pumpkin Seed Corn Muffins: *Toss 1/2 cup shelled pumpkin seeds into the flour mixture before adding it to the batter.*

Toasted Pine Nut Corn Muffins: *Toss 1/2 cup toasted pine nuts into the flour mixture before adding it to the batter.*

Cranberry Muffins

Makes 12 muffins

For the best cranberry muffins, we've added a little cornmeal for crunch and some orange marmalade to balance the sugar. Fresh cranberries, by the way, freeze terrifically well—buy a few packages in the autumn and squirrel them away in your freezer for the next year. If you use frozen cranberries, don't thaw them before chopping or baking; use them straight from the freezer.

Nonstick spray or paper muffin cups
2 cups all-purpose flour
$3/4$ cup sugar
$1/4$ cup yellow or white cornmeal
2 teaspoons baking powder
1 teaspoon baking soda
$1/2$ teaspoon salt
1 cup whole cranberries, fresh or frozen
1 tablespoon grated orange zest
1 large egg, lightly beaten, at room temperature
$3/4$ cup milk (whole, low-fat, or nonfat)
$1/4$ cup sour cream (regular, low-fat, or nonfat)
$1/4$ cup canola or vegetable oil
$1/4$ cup orange marmalade

1. Position the rack in the center of the oven and preheat the oven to 400°F. To prepare the muffin tins, spray the indentations and the rims around them with nonstick spray, or line the indentations with paper muffin cups. If using silicon muffin tins, spray as directed, then place them on a baking sheet.

2. Whisk the flour, $1/2$ cup of the sugar, the cornmeal, baking powder, baking soda, and salt in a medium bowl until uniform. Set aside.

3. Place the cranberries, orange zest, and the remaining $1/4$ cup of sugar in a food processor fitted with the chopping blade or a wide-canister blender. Process or blend for 10 seconds until the mixture resembles cornmeal—do not allow it to become a paste. Scrape the mixture into a large bowl; stir in the egg, milk, sour cream, oil, and marmalade until uniform and smooth. Stir in the flour mixture until moistened.

4. Fill the prepared tins three-quarters full. Use additional greased tins or small, oven-safe, greased ramekins for any leftover batter, or reserve the batter for a second baking. Bake for 25 minutes, or until the muffins have lightly browned, slightly rounded tops. A toothpick inserted in the center of one muffin should come out with a crumb or two attached.

5. Set the pan on a wire rack to cool for 10 minutes. Gently rock each muffin back and forth to release it. Remove the muffins from the pan and cool for 5 minutes more on the rack before serving. If storing or freezing the muffins, cool them completely before sealing in an airtight container or in freezer-safe plastic bags. The muffins will stay fresh for up to 24 hours at room temperature or up to 2 months in the freezer.

> **Cranberry Apple Crunch Muffins:** *Add 3/4 cup chopped dried apple with the marmalade. Top the muffins with Cinnamon Sugar Topping (page 225) before baking.*
>
> **Cranberry Pecan Muffins:** *Add 3/4 cup chopped pecans with the marmalade.*
>
> **Cranberry Walnut Muffins:** *Substitute walnut oil for the canola oil. Add 1/2 cup chopped, toasted walnuts with the marmalade.*
>
> **Spiced Cranberry Date Muffins:** *Add 1 teaspoon ground cinnamon, 1/4 teaspoon ground cloves, and 1/4 teaspoon grated nutmeg with the flour. Add 2/3 cup chopped, pitted dates with the marmalade.*

Cream Cheese Muffins

Makes 12 muffins

These decadent muffins have all the ingredients of a cheesecake, but not the dense, heavy texture. Instead, they have a light, coarse crumb, infused with the tangy taste of cream cheese. They make a splendid addition to any breakfast, brunch, or dessert table. Serve them with plenty of strawberry jam.

Nonstick spray or paper muffin cups
2 cups all-purpose flour
2 teaspoons baking soda
1 teaspoon baking powder
$1/2$ teaspoon salt
4 ounces cream cheese (regular or low-fat, but not nonfat), softened
$1/2$ cup sugar
2 large eggs, at room temperature
8 tablespoons (1 stick) unsalted butter, at room temperature
1 tablespoon lemon juice
2 teaspoons vanilla extract
$2/3$ cup milk (whole, low-fat, or nonfat)

1. Position the rack in the center of the oven and preheat the oven to 400°F. To prepare the muffin tins, spray the indentations and the rims around them with nonstick spray, or line the indentations with paper muffin cups. If using silicon muffin tins, spray as directed, then place them on a baking sheet.

2. Whisk the flour, baking soda, baking powder, and salt in a medium bowl until uniform. Set aside.

3. Place the cream cheese and sugar in the large bowl. Beat with an electric mixer at medium speed for 2 minutes, or until smooth and light. Beat in the eggs one at a time, beating well after each addition. Then beat in the butter, lemon juice, and vanilla until smooth. Reduce the mixer speed to low and slowly pour in the milk. Beat 1 minute or until creamy and smooth.

4. Stir in the prepared flour mixture with a wooden spoon until moistened.

5. Fill the prepared tins three-quarters full. Use additional greased tins or small, oven-safe, greased ramekins for any leftover batter, or reserve the batter for a second baking. Bake for 20 minutes, or until the muffins are lightly browned and a toothpick inserted in the center of one muffin comes out clean.

6. Set the pan on a wire rack to cool for 10 minutes. Gently rock each muffin back and forth to release it. Remove the muffins from the pan and cool for 5 minutes more on the rack before serving. If storing or freezing the muffins, cool them completely before sealing in an airtight container or in freezer-safe plastic bags. The muffins will stay fresh for 48 hours at room temperature or up to 2 months in the freezer.

> **Cream Cheese and Chives Muffins:** *Reduce the sugar to 1/3 cup. Add 3 tablespoons chopped fresh chives with the sugar.*
>
> **Cream Cheese and Jelly Muffins:** *Fill the muffin tins half way with batter, gently spreading it to the rims. Add 1 teaspoon jelly or jam to each muffin, then top with the remaining batter.*
>
> **Cream Cheese and Lox Muffins:** *Reduce the sugar to 1/4 cup. Fold 1/3 cup finely chopped lox into the batter after the milk has been beaten in.*
>
> **Cream Cheese and Olive Muffins:** *Add 1/3 cup finely chopped pitted green olives to the batter after the milk has been beaten in.*
>
> **Cream Cheese Walnut and Raisin Muffins:** *Stir 1/3 cup chopped walnuts and 1/3 cup chopped raisins into the batter after the milk has been beaten in.*

Daiquiri Muffins

Makes 12 muffins

Stirred, not shaken. That's the course for these muffins, an adaptation of the Caribbean drink made of rum, lime juice, and sugar. To get the most juice out of fresh limes, make sure they're at room temperature, roll them along the counter under your palm before cutting them, then use a small reamer or juicer, not a large one more suited to oranges and grapefruits.

Nonstick spray or paper muffin cups
2^1/4 cups all-purpose flour
1 cup plus 1 tablespoon sugar
2 teaspoons baking powder
^{1}/2 teaspoon salt
2 large eggs, at room temperature
8 tablespoons (1 stick) unsalted butter, melted and cooled
^{1}/2 cup yogurt (regular, low-fat, or nonfat)
^{1}/3 cup white or gold rum (do not use dark rum)
^{1}/3 cup lime juice (juice from about 2 large limes)
1 tablespoon grated lime zest (from about 2 large limes)

1. Position the rack in the center of the oven and preheat the oven to 400°F. To prepare the muffin tins, spray the indentations and the rims around them with nonstick spray, or line the indentations with paper muffin cups. If using silicon muffin tins, spray as directed, then place them on a baking sheet.

2. Whisk the flour, 1 cup of the sugar, the baking powder, and salt in a medium bowl until well blended. Set aside.

3. Lightly whisk the eggs in a large bowl, then whisk in the melted butter, yogurt, rum, lime juice, and lime zest until smooth. Use a wooden spoon to stir in the flour mixture until moistened.

4. Fill the prepared tins three-quarters full. Use additional greased tins or small, oven-safe, greased ramekins for any leftover batter, or reserve the batter for a second baking. Use the remaining 1 tablespoon of sugar to dust the tops of the unbaked muffins with a light coating of sugar. Bake for 23 minutes, or until the muffins have

rounded, lightly browned, cracked tops and a toothpick inserted in the center of one muffin comes out with a few moist crumbs attached.

5. Set the pan on a wire rack to cool for 10 minutes. Gently rock each muffin back and forth to release it. Remove the muffins from the pan and cool for 5 minutes more on the rack before serving. If storing or freezing the muffins, cool them completely before sealing in an airtight container or in freezer-safe plastic bags. The muffins will stay fresh for up to 24 hours at room temperature or up to 1 month in the freezer.

Apple Daiquiri Muffins: *Substitute spiced rum for the white or gold rum. Add 1/2 teaspoon ground cinnamon with the salt. Stir 3/4 cup chopped dried apple into the batter just before adding the dry ingredients.*

Banana Daiquiri Muffins: *Add 3/4 cup chopped dried banana to the batter before mixing in the dry ingredients.*

Cherry Daiquiri Muffins: *Add 3/4 cup dried cherries to the batter before mixing in the dry ingredients.*

Cosmopolitan Muffins: *Substitute vodka for the rum. Reduce the lime juice to 1/4 cup. Add 1 1/2 tablespoons frozen cranberry juice concentrate, thawed, with the remaining lime juice.*

Gimlet Muffins: *Substitute vodka for the rum.*

Date Muffins

Makes 12 muffins

Remember that old-fashioned date nut bread, the one that was baked in an empty tin can? These muffins capture that taste—without the worry of baking in tin! Of course, just like date nut bread, the muffins are tastiest when spread with cream cheese.

   1 cup milk (whole, low-fat, or nonfat)

   1^1/2 cups chopped pitted dates

   4 tablespoons (^{1}/2 stick) unsalted butter, cut into ^{1}/2-inch pieces, at room temperature

   3 tablespoons unsulphured molasses

   Nonstick spray or paper muffin cups

   1^1/2 cups all-purpose flour

   ^{1}/2 cup whole wheat flour

   ^{1}/2 cup sugar

   1 tablespoon baking powder

   ^{1}/2 teaspoon ground cinnamon

   ^{1}/2 teaspoon salt

   ^{3}/4 cup chopped, toasted walnut pieces (see page 69 for instructions on toasting walnuts)

   1 large egg, lightly beaten, at room temperature

   2 teaspoons vanilla extract

1. Heat the milk in a small saucepan set over medium heat until small bubbles appear around the pan's rim. Do not boil. Remove from the heat and cool for 2 minutes. Place the dates, butter, and molasses in a large bowl. Pour in the warm milk; stir until the butter melts. Set aside for 10 minutes.

2. Position the rack in the center of the oven and preheat the oven to 400°F. To prepare the muffin tins, spray the indentations and the rims around them with nonstick spray, or line the indentations with paper muffin cups. If using silicon muffin tins, spray as directed, then place them on a baking sheet.

3. Meanwhile, whisk the all-purpose flour, whole wheat flour, sugar, baking powder, cinnamon, and salt in a medium bowl until well blended. Stir in the walnuts. Set aside.

4. Stir the egg and vanilla into the cooled milk mixture. Quickly stir in the prepared dry ingredients until moistened.

5. Fill the prepared tins three-quarters full. Use additional greased tins or small, oven-safe, greased ramekins for any leftover batter, or reserve the batter for a second baking. Bake for 18 minutes, or until the muffins have rounded cracked tops. A toothpick inserted in the center of one muffin should come out with a crumb or two attached.

6. Set the pan on a wire rack to cool for 10 minutes. Gently rock each muffin back and forth to release it. Remove the muffins from the pan and cool for 5 minutes more on the rack before serving. If storing or freezing the muffins, cool them completely before sealing in an airtight container or in freezer-safe plastic bags. The muffins will stay fresh for up to 2 days at room temperature or up to 2 months in the freezer.

Cinnamon Date Muffins: *Top the muffins with Cinnamon Sugar Topping (page 225) before baking.*

Date Brandy Muffins: *Reduce the milk to 2/3 cup. Stir in 1/3 cup brandy with the egg.*

Orange Date Muffins: *Reduce the dates to 1 cup. Add 1/4 cup finely chopped candied orange rind with the egg.*

Raisin Date Muffins: *Reduce dates to 3/4 cup. Add 3/4 cup raisins with remaining dates.*

Earl Grey Tea Muffins

Makes 12 muffins

Earl Grey tea is named for Charles Grey, a British earl, legendary tea-drinker, and prime minister under George IV. The Earl claimed to have gotten his tea recipe from a Chinese servant who introduced him to the bergamot, a small, bitter orange, the peel of which lends its oil to the tea for its characteristic flavor. Steeping this classic tea in warm milk gives these muffins that same perfume. A little oat flour makes them slightly chewy, a nice contrast to that flavor long favored by tea drinkers.

> 1 cup whole milk
> 3 tablespoons loose Earl Grey tea leaves, or 6 Earl Grey tea bags
> Nonstick spray or paper muffin cups
> 1³/4 cups all-purpose flour
> ¹/2 cup oat flour
> ¹/2 cup sugar
> 2 teaspoons baking soda
> 1 teaspoon baking powder
> ¹/2 teaspoon salt
> 1 large egg, at room temperature
> 6 tablespoons (³/4 stick) unsalted butter, melted and cooled
> ¹/2 cup yogurt (regular or low-fat, but not nonfat)
> ¹/4 cup honey

1. Heat the milk in a small pan set over medium heat until small bubbles form around the pan's rim. Do not boil. Remove from the heat, and stir in the tea leaves or submerge the tea bags in the warm milk. Cover the pan and set aside for 45 minutes to steep.

2. Position the rack in the center of the oven and preheat the oven to 400°F. To prepare the muffin tins, spray the indentations and the rims around them with nonstick spray, or line the indentations with paper muffin cups. If using silicon muffin tins, spray as directed, then place them on a baking sheet.

3. Whisk the all-purpose flour, oat flour, sugar, baking soda, baking powder, and salt in a medium bowl until well combined. Set aside.

4. In a large bowl, lightly beat the egg with a whisk; then whisk in the melted butter, yogurt, and honey until well blended. If using loose tea, strain the milk into the bowl, using a fine-mesh strainer, a chinoise, or a large-holed strainer lined with cheesecloth or a double thickness of paper towels. If using tea bags, discard them, then pour the milk into the egg mixture. Stir well with a wooden spoon until smooth, then quickly stir in the prepared flour mixture until moistened.

5. Fill the prepared tins three-quarters full. Use additional greased tins or small, oven-safe, greased ramekins for any leftover batter, or reserve the batter for a second baking. Bake for 25 minutes, or until the muffins are lightly brown, with rounded, cracked tops. A toothpick inserted in the center of one muffin should come out almost clean.

6. Set the pan on a wire rack to cool for 10 minutes. Gently rock each muffin back and forth to release it. Remove the muffins from the pan and cool for 5 minutes more on the rack before serving. If storing or freezing the muffins, cool them completely before sealing in an airtight container or in freezer-safe plastic bags. The muffins will stay fresh for up to 24 hours at room temperature or up to 2 months in the freezer.

Date Tea Muffins: *Mix 3/4 cup chopped pitted dates into the batter just before adding the dry ingredients.*

English Breakfast Tea Muffins: *Substitute English breakfast tea for the Earl Grey tea.*

Jam and Tea Muffins: *Spoon about 2 tablespoons of the prepared batter into the muffin tins, until they are a third full; spread gently to the sides of the tins. Add 1 teaspoon jam or marmalade on top of the batter in each tin. Spoon the remaining batter equally over the tops of the muffins, covering the filling.*

Lemon Tea Muffins: *Use lemon yogurt instead of plain yogurt.*

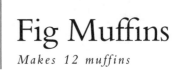

Fig Muffins

Makes 12 muffins

Fresh figs are too wet to make good muffins—but dried figs won't weigh down the batter. Steep the dried figs in warm milk so that the batter will be infused with their taste. Look for plump dried figs, not desiccated or shriveled. The muffins get their texture from whole wheat flour and honey, a classic combination.

8 ounces dried figs, stemmed and chopped (about 1^3/4 cups dried figs)
1 cup whole milk
^{1}/4 cup honey
Nonstick spray or paper muffin cups
1^1/2 cups all-purpose flour
^{1}/2 cup whole wheat flour
^{1}/2 cup sugar
2 teaspoons baking soda
^{1}/2 teaspoon baking powder
^{1}/2 teaspoon salt
1 large egg, at room temperature
^{1}/4 cup canola or vegetable oil
1 tablespoon lemon juice
2 teaspoons vanilla extract

1. Combine the figs, milk, and honey in a small saucepan set over low heat. Heat until small bubbles appear around the pan's rim. Do not boil. Remove from the heat, cover, and steep for 15 minutes, or until the figs are soft and the milk has cooled to room temperature.

2. Meanwhile, position the rack in the center of the oven and preheat the oven to 400°F. To prepare the muffin tins, spray the indentations and the rims around them with nonstick spray, or line the indentations with paper muffin cups. If using silicon muffin tins, spray as directed, then place them on a baking sheet.

3. Whisk the all-purpose flour, whole wheat flour, sugar, baking soda, baking powder, and salt in a medium bowl until uniform. Set aside.

4. In a large bowl, whisk the egg until lightly beaten; whisk in the oil, lemon juice, and vanilla extract until well blended. Pour in the milk, honey, and figs; stir to incorporate. Then stir in the prepared flour mixture until combined.

5. Fill the prepared tins three-quarters full. Use additional greased tins or small, oven-safe, greased ramekins for any leftover batter, or reserve the batter for a second baking. Bake for 16 minutes, or until the muffins are firm and rounded. A toothpick inserted in the center of one muffin should come out clean, provided the figs don't gum up the tester.

6. Set the pan on a wire rack to cool for 10 minutes. Gently rock each muffin back and forth to release it. Remove the muffins from the pan and cool for 5 minutes more on the rack before serving. If storing or freezing the muffins, cool them completely before sealing in an airtight container or in freezer-safe plastic bags. The muffins will stay fresh for up to 24 hours at room temperature or up to 1 month in the freezer.

> **Fig Almond Muffins:** *Substitute almond oil for the canola oil. Add 1/2 cup toasted sliced almonds with the milk mixture.*
>
> **Fig Cinnamon Crunch Muffins:** *Top the muffins with Cinnamon Sugar Topping (page 225) before baking.*
>
> **Fig Lemon Glazed Muffins:** *Top the cooled muffins with Lemon Drizzle (page 227).*
>
> **Fig Maple Muffins:** *Substitute maple syrup for the honey.*
>
> **Fig Nut Crunch Muffins:** *Top the muffins with Nut Crunch Topping (page 229) before baking.*
>
> **Fig Vanilla Glazed Muffins:** *Coat the cooled muffins with Vanilla Dip (page 231).*
>
> **Fig Walnut Muffins:** *Substitute walnut oil for the canola oil. Add 1/2 cup chopped toasted walnuts with the milk mixture.*

Fruitcake Muffins

Makes 12 muffins

Fruitcake is a love-it-or-leave-it proposition. If you're in the latter camp, pass on. But if you're one of those devotees who understands the pleasure of moist, dense fruitcake served at the holidays, these muffins might be just what you've been looking for—with one difference: they're quite light, thanks to the beaten egg whites, which give the batter a lift. But they still have a cakelike crumb, thanks to beating the sugar into the yolks.

Nonstick spray or paper muffin cups
$^1/_2$ cup chopped glacéed cherries
$^1/_4$ cup dried currants
$^1/_4$ cup chopped dried apricots
$^1/_2$ cup brandy
$2^1/_4$ cups all-purpose flour
2 teaspoons baking soda
1 teaspoon baking powder
1 teaspoon salt
$^1/_2$ teaspoon ground ginger
$^1/_2$ teaspoon ground allspice
2 large eggs, separated, at room temperature
$^1/_2$ cup sugar
$^3/_4$ cup buttermilk (regular or low-fat)
10 tablespoons ($1^1/_4$ sticks) unsalted butter, melted and cooled
$^1/_3$ cup unsulphured molasses
1 teaspoon vanilla extract
$^1/_2$ cup chopped toasted pecans

1. Position the rack in the center of the oven and preheat the oven to 400°F. To prepare the muffin tins, spray the indentations and the rims around them with nonstick spray, or line the indentations with paper muffin cups. If using silicon muffin tins, spray as directed, then place them on a baking sheet.

2. Combine the cherries, currants, apricots, and brandy in a small bowl; set aside for 10 minutes.

3. Meanwhile, whisk the flour, baking soda, baking powder, salt, ginger, and allspice in a medium bowl until well combined. Set aside.

4. Place the egg whites in a second medium bowl that is clean and dry. Beat with an electric mixture at high speed until soft peaks form, about 3 minutes. Set aside as well.

5. In a large bowl, whisk the egg yolks just until lightly beaten; then add the sugar and continue whisking until the mixture is thick and sunny yellow, about 3 minutes. Whisk in the buttermilk, melted butter, molasses, and vanilla extract until smooth.

6. Using a wooden spoon, stir in the fruit and any remaining rum into the egg yolk mixture, then stir in the pecans until well distributed. Stir in the flour mixture until incorporated. Then gently fold in the beaten egg whites until no streaks of white are visible.

7. Fill the prepared tins three-quarters full. Use additional greased tins or small, oven-safe, greased ramekins for any leftover batter, or reserve the batter for a second baking. Bake for 20 minutes, or until the muffins are light brown, with firm, rounded tops. A toothpick inserted into the center of one muffin should come out clean.

8. Set the pan on a wire rack to cool for 10 minutes. Gently rock each muffin back and forth to release it. Remove the muffins from the pan and cool for 5 minutes more on the rack before serving. If storing or freezing the muffins, cool them completely before sealing in an airtight container or in freezer-safe plastic bags. The muffins will stay fresh for up to 2 days at room temperature or up to 3 months in the freezer.

Honey Fruitcake Muffins: *Substitute 1/3 cup honey for the molasses.*

Island Fruitcake Muffins: *Substitute coconut rum for the brandy and chopped toasted unsalted cashews for the pecans.*

Rum Raisin Fruitcake Muffins: *Use white or gold rum instead of brandy. Omit the glacéed cherries, currants, and dried apricots; use 1 cup raisins instead.*

Fudge Muffins

Makes 12 muffins

These treats look like muffins, smell like brownies, and taste like heaven. Their dark, heavy, cracked tops almost collapse under the weight of so much fudgy chocolate. They'll stay moist for a few days, long enough to make it on a car trip or in a care package for kids at school or camp.

Nonstick spray or paper muffin cups
8 tablespoons (1 stick) unsalted butter, cut into small pieces
5 ounces semisweet chocolate, chopped; or 5 ounces semisweet chocolate chips
4 ounces unsweetened chocolate, chopped
1^1/2 cups all-purpose flour
2 teaspoons baking soda
^{1}/2 teaspoon salt
1 large egg, at room temperature
1 large egg yolk, at room temperature
1 cup sugar
^{1}/2 cup sour cream (regular or low-fat, but not nonfat)
1 teaspoon vanilla extract

1. Position the rack in the center of the oven and preheat the oven to 400°F. To prepare the muffin tins, spray the indentations and the rims around them with nonstick spray, or line the indentations with paper muffin cups. If using silicon muffin tins, spray as directed, then place them on a baking sheet.

2. Place the butter and both kinds of chocolate in the top of a double boiler set over simmering water. If you don't have a double boiler, place the butter and both kinds of chocolate in a heat-safe bowl that fits snugly over a small pot of simmering water. Stir constantly until half the butter and chocolate is melted. Remove the top of the double boiler or the bowl from the pot; then continue stirring, away from the heat, until the mixture is smooth. Cool for 10 minutes.

3. Meanwhile, whisk the flour, baking soda, and salt in a small bowl until uniform. Set aside.

4. Whisk the egg, egg yolk, and sugar in a large bowl until pale yellow and light, about 2 minutes. Slowly whisk in the chocolate mixture; continue whisking until smooth. Whisk in the sour cream until no traces of white remain. Using a wooden spoon, stir in the vanilla, then stir in the flour mixture until moistened.

5. Fill the prepared tins three-quarters full. Use additional greased tins or small, oven-safe, greased ramekins for any leftover batter, or reserve the batter for a second baking. Bake for 22 minutes, or until the muffins have rounded, cracked tops and a toothpick inserted in the center of one muffin comes out with several moist crumbs attached.

6. Set the pan on a wire rack to cool for 10 minutes. Gently rock each muffin back and forth to release it. Remove the muffins from the pan and cool them for 5 minutes more on the rack before serving. If storing or freezing the muffins, cool them completely before sealing in an airtight container or in freezer-safe plastic bags. The muffins will stay fresh for up to 2 days at room temperature or up to 2 months in the freezer.

> **Cherry Fudge Muffins:** *Add 1/2 cup dried cherries with the vanilla.*
>
> **Chocolate Chip Fudge Muffins:** *Add 3 ounces (1/2 cup) semisweet chocolate chips with the vanilla.*
>
> **Cranberry Fudge Muffins:** *Add 1/2 cup dried cranberries with the vanilla.*
>
> **Fudge Nut Muffins:** *Add 1/2 cup finely chopped toasted nuts, such as hazelnuts, pecans, or walnuts, with the vanilla.*
>
> **Mint Fudge Muffins:** *Add 11/2 teaspoons mint extract with the vanilla.*
>
> **Orange Fudge Muffins:** *Add 11/2 teaspoons orange extract or 1/2 teaspoon orange oil with the vanilla.*

Ginger Muffins

Makes 12 muffins

If you're looking for dark Gingerbread Muffins (see page 92), these are not for you. But if you want golden, tender muffins, delicately infused with ginger, you're in the right place. Look for fresh ginger that's firm, not mushy; the beige skin should be papery, not shriveled or blotchy. Peel off that papery skin, then grate it on a ginger board or with the small holes of a box grater.

Nonstick spray or paper muffin cups
2 cups all-purpose flour
$3/4$ cup sugar
1 tablespoon baking powder
$1/2$ teaspoon salt
1 large egg, at room temperature
$1^1/2$ cups milk (whole, low-fat, or nonfat)
5 tablespoons unsalted butter, melted and cooled
2 teaspoons peeled, grated fresh ginger
1 teaspoon ginger juice (see Note)
$1/2$ teaspoon grated lemon zest

1. Position the rack in the center of the oven and preheat the oven to 400°F. To prepare the muffin tins, spray the indentations and the rims around them with nonstick spray, or line the indentations with paper muffin cups. If using silicon muffin tins, spray as directed, then place them on a baking sheet.

2. Whisk the flour, sugar, baking powder, and salt in a medium bowl until uniform. Set aside.

3. In a large bowl, whisk the egg until lightly beaten. Whisk in the milk, melted butter, ginger, ginger juice, and lemon zest until smooth. Using a wooden spoon, stir in the flour mixture until moistened.

4. Fill the prepared tins three-quarters full. Use additional greased tins or small, oven-safe, greased ramekins for any leftover batter, or reserve the batter for a second baking. Bake for 20 minutes, or until the muffins are light brown, with firm, rounded

tops. A toothpick inserted into the center of one muffin should come out with a few moist crumbs attached.

5. Set the pan on a wire rack to cool for 10 minutes. Gently tip each muffin to one side to make sure it isn't stuck. If one is, gently rock it back and forth to release it. Remove the muffins from the pan and cool them for 5 minutes more on the rack before serving. If storing or freezing the muffins, allow them to cool completely before sealing in an airtight container or in freezer-safe plastic bags. The muffins will stay fresh for up to 24 hours at room temperature or up to 1 month in the freezer.

Note: *Bottled ginger juice is available in many supermarkets, either in the spice aisle or near the Tabasco. You can also make your own by squeezing chopped ginger through a garlic press.*

Candied Ginger Muffins: *Add 1/2 cup chopped crystallized ginger with the milk.*

Ginger Banana Muffins: *Add 2/3 cup chopped dried banana with the milk.*

Ginger Cashew Muffins: *Add 1 cup chopped, unsalted cashews with the flour.*

Ginger Chocolate Chip Muffins: *Add 2/3 cup semisweet chocolate chips with the flour.*

Ginger Coconut Muffins: *Add 2/3 cup shredded unsweetened coconut with the flour.*

Ginger Cranberry Muffins: *Roughly chop 1/2 cup fresh cranberries; sprinkle the chopped cranberries on top of each muffin before baking. Gently press on the berries to help them adhere.*

Ginger Nut Crunch Muffins: *Top the muffins with Nut Crunch Topping (page 229) before baking.*

Ginger Raisin Muffins: *Add 1 cup golden raisins with the milk.*

Lemon Glazed Ginger Muffins: *Top the cooled muffins with Lemon Drizzle (page 227).*

Vanilla Glazed Ginger Muffins: *Coat the cooled muffins with Vanilla Dip (page 231).*

Gingerbread Muffins

Makes 12 muffins

Gingerbread is a homey delight—aromatic, hearty, and comforting. The secret is twofold: 1) use fresh spices, not ones that have sat on your shelf for a year or more, and 2) use good molasses—choose an unsulphured brand with a deep, characteristic taste. Ground black pepper may be a surprise here, but it adds a slight, spicy taste to these cakey muffins.

Nonstick spray or paper muffin cups
$2^1/2$ **cups all-purpose flour**
2 teaspoons baking soda
2 teaspoons ground ginger
$1/2$ **teaspoon ground cinnamon**
$1/2$ **teaspoon salt**
$1/4$ **teaspoon ground cloves**
$1/8$ **teaspoon freshly ground black pepper**
2 large eggs, at room temperature
$1/2$ **cup packed light brown sugar**
1 cup buttermilk (regular or low-fat)
$1/2$ **cup canola or vegetable oil**
$1/3$ **cup unsulphured molasses**
1 teaspoon vanilla extract

1. Position the rack in the center of the oven and preheat the oven to 400°F. To prepare the muffin tins, spray the indentations and the rims around them with nonstick spray, or line the indentations with paper muffin cups. If using silicon muffin tins, spray as directed, then place them on a baking sheet.

2. Whisk the flour, baking soda, ginger, cinnamon, salt, cloves, and black pepper in a medium bowl until uniform. Set aside.

3. In a large bowl, whisk the eggs until lightly beaten, then add the brown sugar and whisk until the mixture is pale brown and very thick, about 2 minutes. Whisk in the buttermilk, oil, molasses, and vanilla until smooth.

4. Using a wooden spoon, quickly stir in the prepared flour mixture until incorporated. The batter will be quite stiff and sticky, but do not overbeat.

5. Fill the prepared tins three-quarters full. Use additional greased tins or small, oven-safe, greased ramekins for any leftover batter, or reserve the batter for a second baking. Bake for 22 minutes, or until the muffins have firm, rounded tops with cracks running through them. A toothpick inserted into the center of one muffin should come out with a crumb or two attached.

6. Set the pan on a wire rack to cool for 10 minutes. Gently tip each muffin to one side to make sure it isn't stuck. If one is, gently rock it back and forth to release it. Remove the muffins from the pan and cool them for 5 minutes more on the rack before serving. If storing or freezing the muffins, allow them to cool completely before sealing in an airtight container or in freezer-safe plastic bags. The muffins will stay fresh for up to 2 days at room temperature or up to 2 months in the freezer.

> **Brandy Gingerbread Muffins:** *Drizzle the tops of the each muffin with 2 teaspoons brandy right after you take them out of the oven.*
>
> **Chestnut Gingerbread Muffins:** *Stir 1/2 cup chopped candied chestnuts into the batter just before adding the flour mixture.*
>
> **Chunky Ginger Gingerbread Muffins:** *Stir 1/2 cup chopped crystallized ginger into the batter just before adding the flour mixture.*
>
> **Figgy Gingerbread Muffins:** *Stir 1/4 cup chopped dried figs and 1/4 cup raisins into the batter just before adding the flour mixture.*
>
> **Gingerbread Cinnamon Streusel Muffins:** *Top the muffins with Cinnamon Streusel Topping (page 224) before baking.*
>
> **Orange Gingerbread Muffins:** *Add 1/2 cup chopped candied orange peel with the buttermilk.*

Gluten-Free Berry Muffins

Makes 12 muffins

If you avoid wheat glutens in your diet, or if you know someone who does, these muffins will become an indispensable part of your baking repertoire. Rich and moist, but light and cakey, they're great for breakfast or dessert. And since you can fold in any berry except strawberries, they're endlessly adaptable. For the various flours used, see A Guide to Some Ingredients (page 11).

    Nonstick spray or paper muffin cups
    1 cup plus 1 tablespoon brown rice flour
    $^1/_2$ cup potato starch flour
    $^1/_2$ cup tapioca flour
    $^1/_2$ cup sugar
    2 teaspoons xanthan gum (see Note)
    2 teaspoons gluten-free baking powder
    $^1/_2$ teaspoon salt
    1 pint berries, hulled if necessary (do not use strawberries)
    2 large eggs, separated, at room temperature
    $^3/_4$ cup milk (whole or low-fat, but not nonfat)
    4 tablespoons ($^1/_2$ stick) unsalted butter, melted and cooled
    $^1/_4$ cup yogurt (regular or low-fat, but not nonfat)
    1 teaspoon gluten-free vanilla extract

1. Position the rack in the center of the oven and preheat the oven to 400°F. To prepare the muffin tins, spray the indentations and the rims around them with nonstick spray, or line the indentations with paper muffin cups. If using silicon muffin tins, spray as directed, then place them on a baking sheet.

2. Whisk 1 cup of the brown rice flour, the potato starch flour, tapioca flour, sugar, xanthan gum, baking powder, and salt in a medium bowl until uniform. Set aside.

3. Toss the berries with the remaining 1 tablespoon brown rice flour in a small bowl until well coated. Set aside as well.

4. Place the egg yolks in a large bowl, whisk them lightly, then beat in the milk, melted butter, yogurt, and vanilla until smooth. Stir in the dry ingredients until incorporated. Set aside for 5 minutes.

5. Meanwhile, place the egg whites in a clean, dry, medium bowl; beat with an electric mixer at high speed until stiff but not dry. Use a rubber spatula to fold the beaten whites into the batter until a few white streaks remain. Gently fold in the coated berries, taking care not to mash them into the batter.

6. Fill the prepared tins three-quarters full. Use additional greased tins or small, oven-safe, greased ramekins for any leftover batter, or reserve the batter for a second baking. Bake for 20 minutes, or until the muffins are pale beige and have slightly rounded tops. A toothpick inserted in the center of one muffin should come out clean.

7. Set the pan on a wire rack to cool for 10 minutes. Gently tip each muffin back and forth to make sure it isn't stuck. If one is, gently rock it back and forth to release it. Remove the muffins from the pan and cool them for 5 minutes more on the rack before serving. If storing the muffins, cool them completely before sealing in an airtight container. Because the berries stay whole, we do not recommend freezing these muffins. They will stay fresh for up to 2 days at room temperature.

Note: *Without the traditional glutens associated with baking, these muffins need something to bind the batter. Xanthan is a thickener made from the fermentation of the natural sugars found in corn. In small amounts, it assures that the muffins will hold together when they cool, rather than falling into crumbs. Xanthan gum is found in most health food stores and many gourmet markets.*

> **Gluten-Free Apple Berry Spice Muffins:** *Add 2 teaspoons apple pie spice mix with the brown rice flour. Reduce the berries to 1 cup. Toss 1 cup chopped dried apple with the remaining berries and the brown rice flour.*
>
> **Gluten-Free Berry Daiquiri Muffins:** *Add 1 teaspoon grated lime zest with the vanilla. Sprinkle each muffin with 1/2 teaspoon sugar before baking.*
>
> **Gluten-Free Lemon Berry Muffins:** *Substitute lemon yogurt for the plain yogurt.*

Graham Cracker Muffins

Makes 12 muffins

Although a sweet reminder of our childhoods, graham crackers, when used for baking, have long been relegated to pie crusts. Here's an exciting way to use them—in dense muffins, perfect with a slather of butter, or (for the kid in all of us) Marshmallow Fluff.

Nonstick spray or paper muffins cups
12 whole graham crackers (see Note)
1 cup all-purpose flour
1 tablespoon baking powder
$1/2$ teaspoon salt
1 large egg, at room temperature
$1/3$ cup applesauce
$1/4$ cup honey
1 cup milk (whole or low-fat, but not nonfat)
6 tablespoons ($3/4$ stick) unsalted butter, melted and cooled
1 teaspoon vanilla extract

1. Position the rack in the center of the oven and preheat the oven to 400°F. To prepare the muffin tins, spray the indentations and the rims around them with nonstick spray, or line the indentations with paper muffin cups. If using silicon muffin tins, spray as directed, then place them on a baking sheet.

2. Break up the graham crackers and place them in a food processor fitted with the chopping blade. Process for about 1 minute, stopping to reposition the larger chunks as necessary, until the crackers are pulverized to crumbs. Transfer the crumbs to a medium bowl and whisk in the flour, baking powder, and salt until uniform. Set aside.

3. In a large bowl, whisk the egg until lightly beaten, then whisk in the applesauce and honey until well blended. Whisk in the milk, melted butter, and vanilla until smooth.

4. Stir the flour mixture into the batter using a wooden spoon. Do not overmix— simply moisten the flour, leaving the batter grainy, even with a few lumps.

5. Fill the prepared tins three-quarters full. Use additional greased tins or small, oven-safe, greased ramekins for any leftover batter, or reserve the batter for a second baking. Bake for 18 minutes, or until the muffins have rounded browned tops and a toothpick inserted in the center of one muffin comes out clean.

6. Set the pan on a wire rack to cool for 10 minutes. Gently tip each muffin to one side to make sure it isn't stuck. If one is, gently rock it back and forth to release it. Remove the muffins from the pan and cool them for 5 minutes more on the rack before serving. If storing or freezing the muffins, allow them to cool completely before sealing in an airtight container or in freezer-safe plastic bags. The muffins will stay fresh for up to 24 hours at room temperature or up to 1 month in the freezer.

Note: You can also use 1½ cups purchased graham cracker crumbs. If you do, omit placing them in a food processor, and simply whisk them into the flour mixture as directed.

Chocolate Chip Graham Cracker Muffins: *Add 2/3 cup semisweet chocolate chips with the flour.*

Chocolate Iced Graham Cracker Muffins: *Top the cooled baked muffins with Chocolate Icing (page 223).*

Graham Cracker Chocolate Crunch Muffins: *Top the muffins with Chocolate Crunch Topping (page 222) before baking.*

Graham Cracker Jam Muffins: *Fill each muffin tin one third full, gently smoothing the batter to the tins' rims. Add 1 teaspoon jam, such as strawberry or blackberry, to each muffin tin, then divide the remaining batter equally among the tins, covering the jam completely.*

Graham Cracker Raisin Muffins: *Add 2/3 cup raisins with the flour.*

Graham Cracker Streusel Muffins: *Top the muffins with Cinnamon Streusel Topping (page 224) before baking.*

Vanilla Glazed Graham Cracker Muffins: *Coat each cooled muffin with Vanilla Dip (page 231).*

Haroseth Muffins

Makes 12 muffins

Haroseth is a mixture of nuts, apples, raisins, and sweet wine; it's eaten during the Passover Seder to remind those gathered of the mortar the people of Israel used when they were slaves in Egypt before the Exodus. One evening just before Passover, as we were passing around muffins from a day of testing, our friend Michelle Miller mentioned that in her family, any leftover haroseth was turned into muffins the next day. Always up to a new challenge, we soon figured out a way to re-create those flavorful muffins. We've included a recipe for haroseth here; if you want to use leftovers, you'll need 1 cup, drained of excess liquid.

Vegetable oil for oiling the muffin tins

1/4 cup walnut pieces

3 eggs, separated, at room temperature

1 large Rome, Empire, or Spy apple, peeled, cored, and quartered

2 teaspoons grated lemon zest (zest from about 1 medium lemon)

1/2 teaspoon ground cinnamon

1/2 teaspoon grated, peeled fresh ginger

1/4 cup sweet wine (such as Manischewitz or Mogen David), or sweet vermouth

1/2 cup walnut oil

1 tablespoon lemon juice

1 cup matzo meal

3/4 cup sugar

1/2 teaspoon salt

1. Position the oven rack in the center of the oven. Preheat the oven to 400°F. Brush the muffin tins with vegetable oil and set aside.

2. Place the walnuts on a baking sheet and bake for 5 minutes, or until golden and fragrant, stirring occasionally. Transfer the hot nuts to the bowl of a food processor fitted with the chopping blade; cool, uncovered, for 5 minutes.

3. Meanwhile, place the egg whites in a medium bowl. Beat with an electric mixer at high speed until stiff but not dry. Set aside.

4. Add the apple, lemon zest, cinnamon, and ginger to the food processor. Pulse the machine until the mixture is finely ground. Add the wine and pulse until a coarse paste is formed. Set aside as well.

5. In a large bowl, whisk the egg yolks, walnut oil, and lemon juice until thick, about 1 minute. With a rubber spatula, stir in the prepared apple and walnut mixture (that is, the haroseth), the matzo meal, sugar, and salt until uniformly blended. Then gently fold in the beaten egg whites until no streaks of white are visible.

6. Fill the prepared tins three-quarters full. Use additional oiled tins or small, oven-safe, oiled ramekins for any leftover batter, or reserve the batter for a second baking. Bake for 22 minutes, or until the tops are puffed and lightly browned and a tooth-pick inserted in the center of one muffin comes out with a few moist crumbs attached.

7. Set the pan on a wire rack to cool for 10 minutes. Gently tip each muffin to one side to make sure it isn't stuck. If one is, gently rock it back and forth to release it. Remove the muffins from the pan and cool them for 5 minutes more on the rack before serving. Or cool them completely before sealing in an airtight container. The muffins will stay fresh for up to 24 hours at room temperature. Because of the extra moisture from the apples and wine, we do not recommend freezing these muffins since they don't thaw well.

Hazelnut Muffins

Makes 12 muffins

Hazelnuts, high in protein, calcium, and vitamin E, have been harvested and eaten in Europe for millennia. They were considered a cure-all by some medieval theologians and physicians, prescribed for everything from a dry cough to oily skin. We can't offer such promises for these muffins—but we can vouch for the brilliant aroma of toasted hazelnuts. Here, we've added a chopped apple to balance the hazelnuts' natural dryness. We prefer this muffin the old-fashioned way: with a glass of cold milk.

Nonstick spray or paper muffin cups
1 cup whole hazelnuts
1¹/₂ cups all-purpose flour
¹/₂ cup whole wheat flour
1 tablespoon baking powder
¹/₂ teaspoon salt
1 large egg, at room temperature
¹/₂ cup packed light brown sugar
¹/₂ cup yogurt (regular, low-fat, or nonfat)
1 cup milk (whole, low-fat, or nonfat)
1 teaspoon vanilla extract
1 large sweet apple, such as Red Delicious or Braeburn, peeled

1. Position the rack in the center of the oven and preheat the oven to 400°F. To prepare the muffin tins, spray the indentations and the rims around them with nonstick spray, or line the indentations with paper muffin cups. If using silicon muffin tins, spray as directed, then place them on a baking sheet.

2. Spread the hazelnuts on a baking sheet and place them in the oven for 5 minutes, until lightly browned and very fragrant, stirring occasionally. Remove from the oven and cool for 5 minutes. Wrap the toasted nuts in a clean kitchen towel; gather the towel into a loose bundle, and rub the nuts inside together, using the towel as an abrasive surface to remove the papery hulls. You'll need to open the towel occasionally and pick out any nuts that have lost their hulls. However, when done, a few specks of hull may still adhere to some of the nuts.

3. Coarsely chop 1/2 cup of the nuts and set them aside. Place the remaining 1/2 cup nuts in a food processor fitted with the chopping blade. Process for about 20 seconds or until the nuts are finely ground, like cornmeal—do not process until they become a paste. Transfer the ground nuts to a medium bowl and whisk in the all-purpose flour, whole wheat flour, baking powder, and salt. Set aside.

4. In a large bowl, whisk the egg and sugar until thick and pale brown, about 2 minutes. Whisk in the yogurt until smooth, then whisk in the milk and vanilla extract.

5. Grate the apple into the bowl, using the large holes of a box grater. Add the remaining chopped nuts and stir until the apple and nuts are well combined with the wet ingredients. Use a wooden spoon to stir in the prepared flour mixture, taking care not to overmix, but simply stirring until the flour is evenly distributed.

6. Fill the prepared tins three-quarters full. Use additional greased tins or small, oven-safe, greased ramekins for any leftover batter, or reserve the batter for a second baking. Bake for 20 minutes, or until the muffins are golden brown with rounded tops. A toothpick inserted in the center of one muffin should come out fairly clean with a crumb or two attached.

7. Set the pan on a wire rack to cool for 10 minutes. Gently tip each muffin to one side to make sure it isn't stuck. If one is, gently rock it back and forth to release it. Remove the muffins from the pan and cool them for 5 minutes more on the rack before serving. If storing or freezing the muffins, allow them to cool completely before sealing in an airtight container or in freezer-safe plastic bags. The muffins will stay fresh for up to 24 hours at room temperature or up to 1 month in the freezer.

> **Chocolate Iced Hazelnut Muffins:** *Ice the cooled, baked muffins with Chocolate Icing (page 223).*
>
> **Hazelnut Cherry Muffins:** *Stir in 1/2 cup dried cherries with the shredded apple.*
>
> **Hazelnut Chocolate Chip Muffins:** *Add 1/2 cup milk chocolate or semisweet chocolate chips with the flour.*
>
> **Hazelnut Cinnamon Muffins:** *Top the muffins with Cinnamon Sugar Topping (page 225) before baking.*
>
> **Hazelnut Crumb Muffins:** *Top the muffins with Crumb Topping (page 226) before baking.*

Honey Muffins

Makes 12 muffins

These delicate, sweet muffins come with dozens of variations built into the base recipe because the variety of honey you use will directly influence the taste. Darker honeys such as buckwheat, chestnut, and pine are particularly good; but more delicate flavors such has orange blossom, star thistle, and even clover will be very aromatic. For an excellent selection of honeys, check out health food stores or gourmet markets—or outlets listed in the Source Guide (see page 237). Serve these gems with the best butter you can find.

Nonstick spray or paper muffin cups
$1^3/4$ cups all-purpose flour
$1/2$ cup whole wheat flour
2 teaspoons baking powder
1 teaspoon baking soda
$1/2$ teaspoon salt
$1/4$ teaspoon grated nutmeg
1 large egg, at room temperature
1 cup honey
$3/4$ cup yogurt (regular, low-fat, or nonfat)
$1/2$ cup milk (whole, low-fat, or nonfat)
6 tablespoons ($3/4$ stick) unsalted butter, melted
1 teaspoon vanilla extract

1. Position the rack in the center of the oven and preheat the oven to 400°F. To prepare the muffin tins, spray the indentations and the rims around them with nonstick spray, or line the indentations with paper muffin cups. If using silicon muffin tins, spray as directed, then place them on a baking sheet.

2. Whisk the all-purpose flour, whole wheat flour, baking powder, baking soda, salt, and nutmeg in a medium bowl until uniform. Set aside.

3. In a large bowl, whisk the egg until lightly beaten, then whisk in the honey until the mixture is light and pale, about 1 minute. Whisk in the yogurt until smooth, then whisk in the milk, melted butter, and vanilla. Stir in the flour mixture with a wooden spoon, just until moistened.

4. Fill the prepared tins three-quarters full. Use additional greased tins or small, oven-safe, greased ramekins for any leftover batter, or reserve the batter for a second baking. Bake for 25 minutes, or until the muffins are browned with rounded, cracked tops. A toothpick inserted into the center of one muffin should come out clean.

5. Set the pan on a wire rack to cool for 10 minutes. Gently tip each muffin to one side to make sure it isn't stuck. If one is, gently rock it back and forth to release it. Remove the muffins from the pan and cool them for 5 minutes more on the rack before serving. If storing or freezing the muffins, allow them to cool completely before sealing in an airtight container or in freezer-safe plastic bags. The muffins will stay fresh for up to 2 days at room temperature or up to 3 months in the freezer.

> **Almond Honey Muffins:** *Add 1/2 teaspoon almond extract with the vanilla. Sprinkle 1 teaspoon sliced almonds on top of each muffin before baking.*
>
> **Honey Cake Muffins:** *Omit the whole wheat flour and increase the all-purpose flour to 2 1/4 cups. Substitute canola oil for the butter.*
>
> **Nonfat Honey Muffins:** *Substitute 1/2 cup unsweetened applesauce for the butter. Use only nonfat yogurt and nonfat milk.*
>
> **Nutty Oat Honey Muffins:** *Omit the whole wheat flour. Add 1/2 cup finely chopped rolled oats (not quick-cooking oats) with the all-purpose flour. Sprinkle 2 teaspoons chopped walnuts or pecans on top of each muffin before baking.*

Jalapeño Corn Muffins

Makes 12 muffins

A Texas tradition, these muffins should be made only with a fresh jalapeño, never a canned or pickled one. There's cornmeal in the mix for texture—use yellow, white, or blue cornmeal, depending on your preference. And use care when seeding the jalapeño. Its oils will stick to your hands; you could get a nasty chile burn if you touch your face or rub your eyes before washing up. These muffins are the first choice to serve alongside a bowl of chili.

Nonstick spray or paper muffin cups
$1^1/2$ cups all-purpose flour
2 tablespoons sugar
1 cup yellow, white, or blue cornmeal
$2^1/2$ teaspoons baking soda
$1/2$ teaspoon baking powder
$1/2$ teaspoon salt
2 large eggs
$1^1/3$ cups buttermilk (regular or low-fat)
6 tablespoons ($3/4$ stick) unsalted butter, melted and cooled
$3/4$ cup corn kernels, fresh (see Note), or frozen (do not thaw)
1 large fresh jalapeño, stemmed, seeded, and finely chopped

1. Position the rack in the center of the oven and preheat the oven to 375°F. To prepare the muffin tins, spray the indentations and the rims around them with nonstick spray, or line the indentations with paper muffin cups. If using silicon muffin tins, spray as directed, then place them on a baking sheet.

2. Whisk the flour, sugar, cornmeal, baking soda, baking powder, and salt in a medium bowl until well blended. Set aside.

3. In a large bowl, whisk the eggs, buttermilk, and melted butter until smooth. Add the corn kernels and jalapeño; stir until well distributed. Stir in the prepared flour mixture with a wooden spoon until the cornmeal is distributed throughout the batter.

4. Fill the prepared tins three-quarters full. Use additional greased tins or small, oven-safe, greased ramekins for any leftover batter, or reserve the batter for a second bak-

ing. Bake for 24 minutes, or until the muffins have bumpy, rounded tops and a toothpick inserted in the center of one muffin comes out with a couple crumbs stuck on it.

5. Set the pan on a wire rack to cool for 10 minutes. Gently rock each muffin back and forth to release it from the tin. Remove the muffins from the pan and cool them for 5 minutes more on the rack before serving. If storing or freezing the muffins, cool completely before sealing in an airtight container or in freezer-safe plastic bags. The muffins will stay fresh for up to 24 hours at room temperature or up to 1 month in the freezer.

Note: *Cutting the corncob in half before you slice off the kernels makes the job easier and less messy.*

Black Bean Jalapeño Corn Muffins: *Add 2/3 cup canned black beans, drained and rinsed, with the melted butter.*

Chili Jalapeño Corn Muffins: *Add 2 tablespoons chili powder with the flour.*

Extra Hot Jalapeño Corn Muffins: *Use two jalapeños instead of one.*

Toasted Cumin Jalapeño Corn Muffins: *Add 2 teaspoons toasted cumin seeds with the flour.*

Lemonade Muffins

Makes 12 muffins

These tender muffins get a bright kick from frozen lemonade concentrate, giving them a wonderful, if very sweet, flavor. Don't use sugar-free brands, made with artificial sweeteners, or the muffins won't rise very well.

> **Nonstick spray or paper muffin cups**
> **2^1/4 cups all-purpose flour**
> **^{1}/3 cup sugar**
> **2 teaspoons baking soda**
> **1 teaspoon baking powder**
> **^{1}/2 teaspoon salt**
> **1 large egg, at room temperature**
> **^{1}/4 cup buttermilk (regular or low-fat)**
> **One 12-ounce can frozen lemonade concentrate, thawed**
> **6 tablespoons (^{3}/4 stick) unsalted butter, melted and cooled**
> **1 tablespoon grated lemon zest**

1. Position the rack in the center of the oven and preheat the oven to 400°F. To prepare the muffin tins, spray the indentations and the rims around them with nonstick spray, or line the indentations with paper muffin cups. If using silicon muffin tins, spray as directed, then place them on a baking sheet.

2. Whisk the flour, sugar, baking soda, baking powder, and salt in a medium bowl until well combined. Set aside.

3. In a large bowl, whisk the egg and buttermilk until well blended. Whisk in the lemonade concentrate, melted butter, and lemon zest until smooth. Stir in the prepared flour mixture until moistened—do not overmix.

4. Fill the prepared tins three-quarters full. Use additional greased tins or small, oven-safe, greased ramekins for any leftover batter, or reserve the batter for a second baking. Bake for 18 minutes, or until the muffins have lightly browned, flat tops and a toothpick inserted in the center of one muffin comes out with a crumb or two attached.

5. Set the pan on a wire rack to cool for 10 minutes. Gently rock each muffin back and forth to release it from the tin. Cool them for 5 minutes more on the rack before serving. If storing or freezing the muffins, allow them to cool completely before sealing in an airtight container or in freezer-safe plastic bags. The muffins will stay fresh for up to 24 hours at room temperature or up to 1 month in the freezer.

Lemon Glazed Lemonade Muffins: *Top the cooled muffins with Lemon Drizzle (page 227).*

Limeade Muffins: *Substitute limeade concentrate for the lemonade concentrate and lime zest for the lemon zest.*

Raspberry Lemonade Muffins: *Gently fold 1/2 cup raspberries into the batter just after adding the flour mixture.*

Strawberry Lemonade Muffins: *Hull and thinly slice 8 large strawberries (about 1/2 pint). Add them along with the lemon zest.*

Lemon Poppy Seed Muffins

Makes 12 muffins

Lemon poppy seed muffins are such a classic that we didn't want to give them short-shrift by making them a variation of Lemonade Muffins (page 106). We wanted a very moist and a little tangy muffin that takes full advantage of the earthy sweetness of the poppy seeds. The secret is a touch of cornmeal, which balances the delicate seeds perfectly.

Nonstick spray or paper muffin cups
1³/4 cups all-purpose flour
¹/2 cup yellow cornmeal
¹/2 cup sugar
¹/3 cup poppy seeds (see Note)
2 teaspoons baking soda
1 teaspoon baking powder
¹/2 teaspoon salt
2 large eggs, at room temperature
1 cup buttermilk (regular or low-fat, but not nonfat)
¹/4 cup canola or vegetable oil
¹/2 cup lemon juice
2 tablespoons grated lemon zest
1 teaspoon vanilla extract

1. Position the rack in the center of the oven and preheat the oven to 400°F. To prepare the muffin tins, spray the indentations and the rims around them with nonstick spray, or line the indentations with paper muffin cups. If using silicon muffin tins, spray as directed, then place them on a baking sheet.

2. Whisk the flour, cornmeal, sugar, poppy seeds, baking soda, baking powder, and salt in a medium bowl until uniform. Set aside.

3. In a large bowl, whisk the eggs and buttermilk until smooth. Whisk in the oil, lemon juice, lemon zest, and vanilla until well combined. Stir in the prepared flour mixture until moistened.

4. Fill the prepared tins three-quarters full. Use additional greased tins or small, oven-safe, greased ramekins for any leftover batter, or reserve the batter for a second baking. Bake for 20 minutes, or until the muffins have lightly browned, rounded tops and a toothpick inserted in the center of one muffin comes out with a few moist crumbs attached.

5. Set the pan on a wire rack to cool for 10 minutes. Gently rock each muffin back and forth to release it from the tin. Cool them for 5 minutes more on the rack before serving. If storing or freezing the muffins, allow them to cool completely before sealing in an airtight container or in freezer-safe plastic bags. The muffins will stay fresh for up to 24 hours at room temperature or up to 1 month in the freezer.

Note: *Since they quickly go rancid at room temperature, poppy seeds are best stored in the freezer for up to one year.*

Lemon Poppy Seed Jam Muffins: *Fill the muffin tins one-third full, spreading the batter gently to the rims. Place 1 teaspoon jam on top of the batter in each tin, then divide the remaining batter equally among the tins, covering the jam completely.*

Lime Poppy Seed Muffins: *Substitute lime zest and lime juice for the lemon zest and lemon juice.*

Orange Poppy Seed Muffins: *Substitute orange zest and orange juice for the lemon zest and lemon juice. Reduce the sugar to 1/3 cup and whisk in 1/3 cup orange marmalade with the eggs.*

Reduced-Fat Lemon Poppy Seed Muffins: *Substitute sugar-free applesauce for the oil.*

Whole Wheat Lemon Poppy Seed Muffins: *Substitute whole wheat flour for the cornmeal.*

Low-Fat Banana Muffins

Makes 12 muffins

What could be more comforting than a breakfast of oatmeal topped with sliced bananas and maple syrup? We've captured that taste in these light, fluffy muffins that are perfect for any meal of the day, or for an afternoon snack. For nuttier-tasting muffins, substitute a nut oil, such as walnut or hazelnut, for the canola oil.

Nonstick spray or paper muffin cups
3 large egg whites, at room temperature
1^{1}/$_{2}$ cups all-purpose flour
^{2}/$_{3}$ cup oat flour (see A Guide to Some Ingredients, page 11)
3 tablespoons sugar
2 teaspoons baking soda
^{1}/$_{2}$ teaspoon ground cinnamon
3 large ripe bananas
^{2}/$_{3}$ cup nonfat milk
^{1}/$_{2}$ cup maple syrup, preferably Grade A Dark Amber
^{1}/$_{4}$ cup canola oil or walnut oil
1 teaspoon vanilla extract

1. Position the rack in the center of the oven and preheat the oven to 400°F. To prepare the muffin tins, spray the indentations and the rims around them with nonstick spray, or line the indentations with paper muffin cups. If using silicon muffin tins, spray as directed, then place them on a baking sheet.

2. Beat the egg whites in a medium bowl with an electric mixer at high speed until soft peaks form. Set aside.

3. In a second medium bowl, whisk the all-purpose flour, oat flour, sugar, baking soda, and cinnamon until well blended. Set aside as well.

4. Using a potato masher, mash the bananas in a large bowl until smooth. Alternatively, squeeze the bananas through a potato ricer if they are the slightest bit firm. Using a wooden spoon, stir in the milk, maple syrup, oil, and vanilla. Then stir in the prepared flour mixture until moistened. Gently fold in the egg whites, using long, even

arcs to incorporate them. Continue folding, albeit gently, until no white streaks are visible.

5. Fill the prepared tins three-quarters full. Use additional greased tins or small, oven-safe, greased ramekins for any leftover batter, or reserve the batter for a second baking. Bake for 25 minutes, or until the muffins are lightly browned, have slightly rounded tops, and a toothpick inserted in the center of one muffin comes out with a few moist crumbs attached.

6. Set the pan on a wire rack to cool for 10 minutes. Gently tip each muffin to one side to make sure it isn't stuck. If one is, gently rock the muffin back and forth to release it. Remove the muffins from the pan and cool for 5 minutes more on the rack before serving. If storing or freezing the muffins, cool them completely before sealing in an airtight container or in freezer-safe plastic bags. The muffins will stay fresh for up to 24 hours at room temperature or up to 2 months in the freezer.

Low-Fat Banana Kiwi Muffins: *Peel and chop three medium kiwis. Fold them in after adding the flour mixture.*

Low-Fat Banana Mango Muffins: *Omit the nonfat milk. Add 2/3 cup mango nectar with the maple syrup.*

Low-Fat Banana Orange Muffins: *Add 1 tablespoon grated orange zest with the maple syrup.*

Low-Fat Banana Strawberry Muffins: *Fold in 1 cup thinly sliced, hulled strawberries after adding the flour mixture.*

Low-Fat Banana Streusel Muffins: *Top the muffins with Low-Fat Streusel Topping (page 228) before baking.*

Low-Fat Banana Vanilla Glazed Muffins: *Coat the cooled muffins with Vanilla Dip (page 231).*

Low-Fat Triple Banana Muffins: *Omit the nonfat milk. Add 2/3 cup banana nectar with the maple syrup. Mix 2/3 cup chopped dried banana into the batter after adding the flour mixture.*

Low-Fat Berry Muffins

Makes 12 muffins

This versatile berry muffin may be low in calories, but it's definitely worth its weight in taste and texture—especially with two cups of juicy fruit offset by chewy rolled oats. A touch of vinegar adds tenderness and accents the sweet/tart flavor.

1 cup nonfat milk
3/4 cup rolled oats (do not use quick-cooking oats)
2 teaspoons apple cider vinegar
Nonstick spray or paper muffin cups
1 1/2 cups plus 1 tablespoon all-purpose flour
2 teaspoons baking soda
1/2 teaspoon salt
1 pint berries, hulled if necessary (do not use strawberries)
3/4 cup packed light brown sugar
1/4 cup canola or vegetable oil
1 large egg, lightly beaten, at room temperature
1 teaspoon vanilla extract

1. Combine the milk, oats, and vinegar in a large bowl; stir until well blended. Let the mixture stand undisturbed at room temperature for 20 minutes. The milk will thicken and sour.

2. Position the rack in the center of the oven and preheat the oven to 400°F. To prepare the muffin tins, spray the indentations and the rims around them with nonstick spray, or line the indentations with paper muffin cups. If using silicon muffin tins, spray as directed, then place them on a baking sheet.

3. Whisk 1 1/2 cups all-purpose flour, the baking soda, and salt in a small bowl until well combined. In a second small bowl, mix the berries and the remaining 1 tablespoon flour until the berries are well coated. Set both bowls aside.

4. Using a wooden spoon, stir the brown sugar, oil, egg, and vanilla into the oat mixture until uniform and somewhat smooth. Stir in the flour mixture until moistened. Gently fold in the coated berries, taking care not to break them up.

5. Fill the prepared tins three-quarters full. Use additional greased tins or small, oven-safe, greased ramekins for any leftover batter, or reserve the batter for a second baking. Bake for 25 minutes, or until the muffins are lightly browned with flat, cracked tops. The muffins should be firm to the touch.

6. Set the pan on a wire rack to cool for 10 minutes. Gently tip each muffin to one side to make sure it isn't stuck. If one is, gently rock it back and forth to release it. Remove the muffins from the pan, place them upside down on the wire rack, and cool for 5 minutes more. This stops the muffins from collapsing. Turn them over and serve, or cool them completely before sealing them in an airtight container. They will stay fresh for up to 24 hours at room temperature. Because the berries remain whole, we do not recommend freezing these muffins.

> **Low-Fat Balsamic Black Pepper Berry Muffins:** *Substitute 2 teaspoons balsamic vinegar for the apple cider vinegar; add 1/2 teaspoon ground black pepper with the salt.*
>
> **Low-Fat Lemon Glazed Berry Muffins:** *Top the cooled muffins with Lemon Drizzle (page 227).*
>
> **Low-Fat Orange Berry Muffins:** *Reduce berries to 1 1/2 cups. Toss 1/2 cup chopped, candied orange zest with the remaining berries and the flour.*
>
> **Low-Fat Streusel Crunch Berry Muffins:** *Top the muffins with Low-Fat Streusel Topping (page 228) before baking.*
>
> **Low-Fat Vanilla Glazed Berry Muffins:** *Coat the cooled muffins with Vanilla Dip (page 231).*

Low-Fat Cherry Muffins

Makes 12 muffins

We got rid of most of the fat in these muffins by using canned cherry pie filling. We also added a little bran, which absorbs the excess moisture given off by the pie filling. It's just enough bran to give the crumb some tooth but still keep it surprisingly light.

Nonstick spray or paper muffin cups
1¹/₂ cups all-purpose flour
¹/₂ cup wheat bran (do not use bran cereal)
2 teaspoons baking soda
¹/₂ teaspoon baking powder
¹/₂ teaspoon salt
One 21-ounce can cherry pie filling
¹/₃ cup sugar
1 large egg, lightly beaten, at room temperature
¹/₂ cup nonfat yogurt
2 tablespoons almond oil or vegetable oil
¹/₂ teaspoon almond extract

1. Position the rack in the center of the oven and preheat the oven to 400°F. To prepare the muffin tins, spray the indentations and the rims around them with nonstick spray, or line the indentations with paper muffin cups. If using silicon muffin tins, spray as directed, then place them on a baking sheet.

2. Whisk the flour, bran, baking soda, baking powder, and salt in a medium bowl until uniform. Set aside.

3. Spoon the cherry pie filling into a large bowl; stir in the sugar until dissolved. Then stir in the egg, yogurt, oil, and almond extract until uniform. Finally, stir in the flour mixture until moistened.

4. Fill the prepared tins three-quarters full. Use additional greased tins or small, oven-safe, greased ramekins for any leftover batter, or reserve the batter for a second baking. Bake for 20 minutes, or until the muffins are lightly browned with flat tops and

a toothpick inserted in the center of one muffin comes out with a few moist crumbs attached.

5. Set the pan on a wire rack to cool for 10 minutes. Gently rock each muffin back and forth to release it. Remove the muffins from the pan and cool them for 5 minutes more on the rack before serving. If storing or freezing the muffins, cool them completely before sealing in an airtight container or in freezer-safe plastic bags. The muffins will stay fresh for up to 24 hours at room temperature or up to 2 months in the freezer.

Low-Fat Cherry Ginger Muffins: *Add 1/4 cup finely chopped crystallized ginger with the yogurt.*

Low-Fat Cherry Streusel Muffins: *Top the muffins with Low-Fat Streusel Topping (page 228) before baking.*

Low-Fat Cherry Vanilla Muffins: *Omit the almond extract. Add 2 teaspoons vanilla extract with the yogurt. Coat the cooled muffins with Vanilla Dip (page 231).*

Low-Fat Spiced Cherry Muffins: *Add 1 teaspoon ground cinnamon, 1/2 teaspoon grated nutmeg, and 1/2 teaspoon ground ginger with the salt.*

Low-Fat Chocolate Chip Muffins

Makes 12 muffins

Unsweetened applesauce is a common substitute for some or all of the fat in baking. Its mild taste doesn't assert itself like other substitutes, such as apple butter or lekvar (a prune paste). Instead, the taste of vanilla, brown sugar, and, most important, chocolate chips can come through—as in these low-fat treats which are best warm, right out of the oven.

Nonstick spray or paper muffin cups
1^1/$_4$ cups all-purpose flour
2 teaspoons baking powder
^{1}/$_2$ teaspoon salt
1 large egg, at room temperature
1 large egg white, at room temperature
^{1}/$_2$ cup plus 2 tablespoons packed light brown sugar
^{1}/$_4$ cup unsweetened applesauce
3^1/$_2$ tablespoons canola or vegetable oil
2 teaspoons vanilla extract
^{1}/$_2$ cup semisweet chocolate chips

1. Position the rack in the center of the oven and preheat the oven to 400°F. To prepare the muffin tins, spray the indentations and the rims around them with nonstick spray, or line the indentations with paper muffin cups. If using silicon muffin tins, spray as directed, then place them on a baking sheet.

2. Whisk the flour, baking powder, and salt in a small bowl until uniform. Set aside.

3. Separate the egg, placing the yolk in a large bowl and the white in a medium bowl. Add the second white to the first. Set both whites aside.

4. Lightly beat the yolk with a whisk, then whisk in the brown sugar, applesauce, oil, and vanilla until well blended. Set aside.

5. Beat the whites with an electric mixer at high speed until soft peaks form, about 2 minutes.

6. To assemble the muffins, use a rubber spatula to fold the flour mixture into the egg yolk and brown sugar mixture. Then quickly fold in the beaten egg whites; there should be streaks of white in the batter. Finally, fold in 1/3 cup of the chocolate chips.

7. Fill the prepared tins three-quarters full. Use additional greased tins or small, oven-safe, greased ramekins for any leftover batter, or reserve the batter for a second baking. Sprinkle the remaining chocolate chips equally over the tops of the unbaked muffins. Bake for 22 minutes, or until the muffins are lightly golden brown with rounded tops. A toothpick inserted into the center of one muffin should come out clean.

8. Set the pan on a wire rack to cool for 10 minutes. Gently rock each muffin back and forth to release it. Remove the muffins from the pan and cool them for 5 minutes more on the rack before serving. If storing or freezing the muffins, cool them completely before sealing in an airtight container or in freezer-safe plastic bags. The muffins will stay fresh for up to 2 days at room temperature or up to 2 months in the freezer.

Low-Fat Chocolate Chip Ginger Muffins: *Add 1/4 cup chopped crystallized ginger with the chocolate chips.*

Low-Fat Chocolate Chip Streusel Muffins: *Top the muffins with Low-Fat Streusel Topping (page 228) before baking.*

Low-Fat Mint Chocolate Chip Muffins: *Reduce the vanilla to 1 teaspoon. Add 1 teaspoon mint extract and 5 drops green food coloring with the remaining vanilla.*

Low-Fat Peanut Butter Chocolate Chip Muffins: *Reduce the chocolate chips to 1 1/2 tablespoons. Fold 1/3 cup peanut butter chips into the batter. Divide the remaining chocolate chips on top of each muffin before baking.*

Low-Fat White Chocolate Chip Cherry Muffins: *Substitute 1/2 cup white chocolate chips for the semisweet chips. Fold 1/4 cup dried cherries into the batter with 1/3 cup of the chips. Top the muffins with the remaining white chocolate chips, as directed.*

Low-Fat Corn Muffins

Makes 12 muffins

These muffins have smooth, golden, flat tops; underneath is a moist crumb the belies its low-fat name. Sweetened only with honey, they make wonderful sandwich buns for smoked turkey or low-fat ham—but that's not to say you shouldn't try them on a Sunday morning with eggs, or on a Tuesday night with chili.

Nonstick spray or paper muffin cups
1³/4 cups yellow cornmeal
³/4 cup all-purpose flour
2 teaspoons baking soda
1 teaspoon baking powder
¹/2 teaspoon salt
1 large egg, at room temperature
1¹/2 cups nonfat yogurt
6 tablespoons honey
2 tablespoons canola oil

1. Position the rack in the center of the oven and preheat the oven to 375°F. To prepare the muffin tins, spray the indentations and the rims around them with nonstick spray, or line the indentations with paper muffin cups. If using silicon muffin tins, spray as directed, then place them on a baking sheet.

2. Whisk the cornmeal, flour, baking soda, baking powder, and salt in a medium bowl until uniform. Set aside.

3. In a large bowl, whisk the egg and yogurt until smooth, then whisk in the honey and oil. Using a wooden spoon, stir in the cornmeal mixture, but only until incorporated—the batter should be grainy.

4. Fill the prepared tins three-quarters full. Use additional greased tins or small, oven-safe, greased ramekins for any leftover batter, or reserve the batter for a second baking. Bake for 20 minutes, or until the muffins have lightly browned tops and a toothpick inserted in the center of one muffin comes out clean.

5. Set the pan on a wire rack to cool for 10 minutes. Gently rock each muffin back and forth to release it. Remove the muffins from the pan and cool for 5 minutes more

on the rack before serving. If storing or freezing the muffins, cool them completely before sealing in an airtight container or in freezer-safe plastic bags. The muffins will stay fresh for up to 24 hours at room temperature or up to 1 month in the freezer.

Low-Fat Black Bean Corn Muffins: *Add 1 cup canned black beans, rinsed and drained, with the honey and oil.*

Low-Fat Blueberry Corn Muffins: *Sprinkle 8 fresh blueberries on the top of each muffin before baking (you'll need about 1 pint of blueberries). Gently press the berries into the batter to help them adhere to the muffins as they bake.*

Low-Fat Cranberry Corn Muffins: *Add 3/4 cup dried cranberries with the honey and oil.*

Low-Fat Indian Pudding Corn Muffins: *Substitute unsulphered molasses for the honey. Add 1 teaspoon ground cinnamon and 1/2 teaspoon ground ginger with the salt.*

Low-Fat Pimiento Corn Muffins: *Add one 6-ounce jar pimientos, drained and chopped, with the honey and oil.*

Low-Fat Peach Muffins

Makes 12 muffins

The secret to cutting down on the fat is to use canned peach pie filling. A touch of cornmeal gives these muffins a delicate, toothy crumb, but brown sugar and cinnamon make them taste like peach pie.

Nonstick spray or paper muffin cups
1¹/₄ cups all-purpose flour
¹/₂ cup yellow cornmeal
1 teaspoon baking soda
1 teaspoon baking powder
¹/₂ teaspoon ground cinnamon
¹/₂ teaspoon salt
One 21-ounce can peach pie filling (see Note)
¹/₂ cup packed dark brown sugar
¹/₂ cup nonfat yogurt
2 tablespoons almond oil or canola oil
1 large egg, lightly beaten, at room temperature
1 teaspoon vanilla extract

1. Position the rack in the center of the oven and preheat the oven to 400°F. To prepare the muffin tins, spray the indentations and the rims around them with nonstick spray, or line the indentations with paper muffin cups. If using silicon muffin tins, spray as directed, then place them on a baking sheet.

2. Whisk the flour, cornmeal, baking soda, baking powder, cinnamon, and salt in a medium bowl until uniform. Set aside.

3. Place the pie filling in a large bowl; stir in the brown sugar until dissolved. Stir in the yogurt, oil, egg, and vanilla until smooth. Then stir in the prepared flour mixture, until incorporated.

4. Fill the prepared tins three-quarters full. Use additional greased tins or individual, ovensafe, greased ramekins for any leftover batter, or reserve the batter for a second baking. Bake for 18 minutes, or until the tops are browned and a toothpick inserted in the center of one muffin comes out with a few moist crumbs attached.

5. Set the pan on a wire rack to cool for 10 minutes. Gently tip each muffin to one side to make sure it isn't stuck. If one is, gently rock it back and forth to release it from the tin. Remove the muffins from the pan and cool them for 5 minutes more on the rack before serving. If storing or freezing the muffins, cool them completely before sealing in an airtight container or in freezer-safe plastic bags. The muffins will stay fresh for up to 3 days at room temperature or up to 3 months in the freezer.

Note: *After you've opened the can of pie filling, use a pair of kitchen scissors to cut down into the mixture, thereby cutting the peaches into small bits. You can also use a paring knife, but be careful of your fingers near the open can's rim.*

Low-Fat Peach Almond Muffins: *Substitute almond extract for the vanilla. Sprinkle each muffin with 2 teaspoons sliced almonds before baking.*

Low-Fat Peach Cinnamon Crunch Muffins: *Top the muffins with Cinnamon Sugar Topping (page 225) before baking.*

Low-Fat Peach Streusel Muffins: *Top the muffins with Low-Fat Streusel Topping (page 228) before baking.*

Low-Fat Peach Vanilla Glazed Muffins: *Coat the cooled muffins with Vanilla Dip (page 231).*

Low-Fat Peach Walnut Muffins: *Substitute walnut oil for the almond oil. Add 1/2 cup chopped walnuts with the flour.*

Lychee Muffins

Makes 12 muffins

Lychee muffins may seem a stretch; but lychees, prized for their perfumy aroma and sweet taste, are often folded into rice flour pastries. Unfortunately, fresh lychees are hard to find and even more difficult to pit, but canned lychees are readily available and easy to work with. Look for them in the Asian aisle of your supermarket or in the canned fruit section.

Nonstick spray or paper muffin cups
2 cups all-purpose flour
1 tablespoon baking powder
1/2 teaspoon salt
One 20-ounce can lychees in syrup, drained
1 large egg, lightly beaten, at room temperature
1/2 cup sugar
1/2 cup yogurt (regular, low-fat, or nonfat)
1/4 cup canola or vegetable oil

1. Position the rack in the center of the oven and preheat the oven to 400°F. To prepare the muffin tins, spray the indentations and the rims around them with nonstick spray, or line the indentations with paper muffin cups. If using silicon muffin tins, spray as directed, then place them on a baking sheet.

2. Whisk the flour, baking powder, and salt in a medium bowl until uniform. Set aside.

3. Pour the lychees into a food processor fitted with the chopping blade; add the egg and sugar. Process for 30 seconds or until the mixture is fairly smooth, with perhaps just a few small pieces of lychee left in the mixture.

4. Transfer the lychee purée to a large bowl; whisk in the yogurt and oil until well blended. Stir in the flour mixture with a wooden spoon until moistened.

5. Fill the prepared tins three-quarters full. Use additional greased tins or small, oven-safe, greased ramekins for any leftover batter, or reserve the batter for a second baking. Bake for 22 minutes, or until the tops are rounded and lightly browned and a toothpick inserted in the center of one muffin comes out with a crumb or two attached.

6. Set the pan on a wire rack to cool for 10 minutes. Gently rock each muffin back and forth to release it from the tin. Remove the muffins from the pan and cool them for 5 minutes more on the rack before serving. If storing or freezing the muffins, allow them to cool completely before sealing in an airtight container or in freezer-safe plastic bags. The muffins will stay fresh for up to 2 days at room temperature or up to 2 months in the freezer.

Lychee Chestnut Muffins: *Stir in 2/3 cup chopped candied chestnuts with the yogurt.*

Lychee Coconut Muffins: *Add 1/2 cup unsweetened coconut flakes with the flour.*

Lychee Golden Raisin Muffins: *Add 1/2 cup golden raisins with the flour.*

Lychee Green Tea Muffins: *Add 1 tablespoon powdered green tea (do not use instant green tea) with the flour.*

Lychee Papaya Muffins: *Stir in 3/4 cup chopped dried papaya with the yogurt.*

Macadamia Muffins

Makes 12 muffins

O ne of the oiliest nuts, macadamias are opulent, over-the-top treats. Even better, they bake up sweet and rich in these tender muffins—which must be baked at a lower temperature so that the nuts can slowly release their flavor without scorching.

Nonstick spray or paper muffins cups
1 cup unsalted macadamia nuts
2^1/4 cups all-purpose flour
^{2}/3 cup sugar
^{1}/2 cup shredded sweetened coconut
2 teaspoons baking soda
1 teaspoon baking powder
^{1}/2 teaspoon salt
2 large eggs, at room temperature
1 cup buttermilk (regular or low-fat)
8 tablespoons (1 stick) unsalted butter, melted and cooled
1 teaspoon vanilla extract

1. Position the rack in the center of the oven and preheat the oven to 350°F. To prepare the muffin tins, spray the indentations and the rims around them with nonstick spray, or line the indentations with paper muffin cups. If using silicon muffin tins, spray as directed, then place them on a baking sheet.

2. Place the nuts on a lipped baking sheet and bake for 7 minutes, stirring occasionally, until lightly browned and fragrant. Cool for 10 minutes, then finely chop. Transfer the nuts to a medium bowl and stir in the flour, sugar, coconut, baking soda, baking powder, and salt until well blended. Set aside.

3. In a large bowl, whisk the eggs and buttermilk until smooth. Whisk in the melted butter and vanilla. Gently stir in the flour mixture until the nuts are distributed evenly in the batter. Do not overmix.

4. Fill the prepared tins three-quarters full. Use additional greased tins or small, oven-safe, greased ramekins for any leftover batter, or reserve the batter for a second bak-

ing. Bake for 23 minutes, or until the muffins have rounded, cracked tops and a toothpick inserted in the center of one muffin comes out fairly clean, with just a crumb or two.

5. Set the pan on a wire rack to cool for 10 minutes. Gently rock each muffin back and forth to release and remove it from the tin. Cool them for 5 minutes more on the rack before serving. If storing or freezing the muffins, cool them completely before sealing in an airtight container or in freezer-safe plastic bags. The muffins will stay fresh for up to 2 days at room temperature or up to 2 months in the freezer.

Macadamia Banana Muffins: *Reduce the coconut to 1/4 cup. Add 1/2 cup chopped dried banana with the vanilla.*

Macadamia Carrot Muffins: *Reduce the coconut to 1/4 cup. Add 1/3 cup shredded carrot with the vanilla.*

Macadamia Chocolate Chip Muffins: *Reduce the coconut to 1/4 cup. Add 1/3 cup semisweet chocolate chips with the flour.*

Macadamia Ginger Muffins: *Reduce the coconut to 1/4 cup. Add 1/3 cup chopped crystallized ginger with the remaining coconut.*

Macadamia Pineapple Muffins: *Reduce the coconut to 1/4 cup. Add 1/2 cup chopped dried pineapple with the remaining coconut.*

Macaroon Muffins

Makes 12 muffins

The key ingredient in these dessert muffins is marzipan, available in cans or tubes in most supermarkets. The almond oil adds that extra sweetness to the batter, but you can substitute canola oil in a pinch. Let these muffins cool completely before serving—that way, they get dense and crunchy, like a macaroon cookie.

> **Nonstick spray or paper muffin cups**
> **2 cups all-purpose flour**
> **1 tablespoon baking powder**
> **$^1/_2$ teaspoon salt**
> **One 7-ounce tube marzipan**
> **1 cup sugar**
> **1 large egg, at room temperature**
> **$^3/_4$ cup milk (whole, low-fat, or nonfat)**
> **$^1/_4$ cup almond oil or vegetable oil**
> **$^1/_2$ teaspoon almond extract**

1. Position the rack in the center of the oven and preheat the oven to 375°F. To prepare the muffin tins, spray the indentations and the rims around them with nonstick spray, or line the indentations with paper muffin cups. If using silicon muffin tins, spray as directed, then place them on a baking sheet.

2. Whisk the flour, baking powder, and salt in a large bowl until uniform. Set aside.

3. Cut the marzipan into 1-inch pieces and place them in a food processor fitted with the chopping blade. Add the sugar, then pulse on and off until the mixture has a grainy consistency. Add the egg and process for 20 seconds or until the mixture first forms a paste, then turns into a ball. With the machine running, pour the milk in a slow stream through the feed tube, then pour in the oil and almond extract. Process 1 minute or until a thick, smooth paste is formed.

4. Add the paste to the prepared flour mixture and stir just until the flour is incorporated throughout. Do not overmix.

5. Fill the prepared tins three-quarters full. Use additional greased tins or small, oven-safe, greased ramekins for any leftover batter, or reserve the batter for a second bak-

ing. Bake for 16 minutes, or until the tops are smooth and lightly browned and a toothpick inserted in the center of one muffin comes out with a few moist crumbs attached.

6. Set the pan on a wire rack to cool for 10 minutes. Gently rock each muffin back and forth to release and remove it from the tin. To assure the right texture, cool them for 30 minutes more on the rack before serving. If storing or freezing the muffins, cool them completely before sealing in an airtight container or in freezer-safe plastic bags. The muffins will stay fresh for up to 24 hours at room temperature or up to 1 month in the freezer.

> **Apricot Macaroon Muffins:** *Fill the muffin tins one-third full, gently spreading the batter to the rims. Place 1 teaspoon apricot jam on top of each muffin, then divide the remaining batter equally among the tins, covering the jam completely.*
>
> **Cinnamon Crunch Macaroon Muffins:** *Top the muffins with Cinnamon Sugar Topping (page 225) before baking.*
>
> **Cinnamon Macaroon Muffins:** *Add 1 teaspoon ground cinnamon with the flour.*
>
> **Cranberry Macaroon Muffins:** *Add 3/4 cup dried cranberries with the flour.*
>
> **Ginger Macaroon Muffins:** *Add 1 teaspoon ground ginger with the flour.*
>
> **Lemon Macaroon Muffins:** *Add 2 teaspoons grated lemon zest with the egg.*
>
> **Nutmeg Macaroon Muffins:** *Add 1/2 teaspoon grated nutmeg with the flour.*

Maple Muffins

Makes 12 muffins

Look no further for the perfect breakfast, a cross between pancakes and muffins. There's no better way to serve these than hot out of the oven, slathered in butter.

Nonstick spray or paper muffin cups
2 cups all-purpose flour
1 tablespoon baking powder
^{1}/2 teaspoon salt
2 large eggs, at room temperature
^{1}/2 cup maple syrup, preferably Grade A Dark Amber
3 tablespoons maple sugar (see A Guide to Some Ingredients, page 11)
^{3}/4 cup milk (whole, low-fat, or nonfat)
4 tablespoons (^{1}/2 stick) unsalted butter, melted and cooled
1 teaspoon vanilla extract
^{1}/4 teaspoon apple cider vinegar

1. Position the rack in the center of the oven and preheat the oven to 400°F. To prepare the muffin tins, spray the indentations and the rims around them with nonstick spray, or line the indentations with paper muffin cups. If using silicon muffin tins, spray as directed, then place them on a baking sheet.

2. Whisk the flour, baking powder, and salt in a medium bowl until well combined. Set aside.

3. In a large bowl, whisk the eggs until lightly beaten. Whisk in the maple syrup and maple sugar; continue whisking until thick and pale brown, about 1 minute. Whisk in the milk, melted butter, vanilla, and vinegar. Finally, use a wooden spoon to stir in the prepared flour mixture until moistened.

4. Fill the prepared tins three-quarters full. Use additional greased tins or small, oven-safe, greased ramekins for any leftover batter, or reserve the batter for a second baking. Bake for 20 minutes, or until the muffins are golden with rounded, cracked tops. A toothpick inserted into the center of one muffin should come out with a crumb or two attached.

5. Set the pan on a wire rack to cool for 10 minutes. Gently rock each muffin back and forth to release and remove it from the tin. Cool them for 5 minutes more on the rack before serving. If storing or freezing the muffins, cool them completely before sealing in an airtight container or in freezer-safe plastic bags. The muffins will stay fresh for up to 24 hours at room temperature or up to 1 month in the freezer.

Granola Maple Muffins: *Sprinkle 2 teaspoons granola on top of each muffin before baking.*

Maple Cinnamon Crunch Muffins: *Top the muffins with Cinnamon Sugar Topping (page 225) before baking.*

Maple Rum Currant Muffins: *Omit the vinegar. Add 1 teaspoon rum extract with the vanilla. Mix 1/2 cup dried currants in with the maple syrup.*

Spiced Apricot Maple Muffins: *Omit the vinegar. Add 1 teaspoon ground cinnamon and 1/2 teaspoon grated nutmeg with the salt. Fill the tins one-third full, gently spreading the batter to the rims. Place 1 drained, canned apricot half on top, then divide the remaining batter equally among the tins, covering the apricot half completely.*

Margarita Muffins

Makes 12 muffins

High quality tequila will help these south-of-the-border muffins taste just like the cocktail they're named for. Serve them with huevos rancheros for a festive, Mexican-style breakfast. Coarse salt, such as kosher salt, gives the topping a little bite, much like a margarita gets from a salt-rimmed glass—but it's entirely optional.

Nonstick spray or paper muffin cups
2 cups all-purpose flour
$^3/_4$ cup sugar
$^1/_4$ cup yellow or blue cornmeal
2 teaspoons baking soda
$^1/_2$ teaspoon fine salt
1 large egg, at room temperature
$^1/_2$ cup sour cream (regular or low-fat, but not nonfat)
$^1/_2$ cup tequila
$^1/_3$ cup orange juice
$^1/_4$ cup canola or vegetable oil
$^1/_4$ cup lime juice
$1^1/_2$ teaspoons grated lime zest
$1^1/_2$ teaspoons coarse salt (optional)

1. Position the rack in the center of the oven and preheat the oven to 400°F. To prepare the muffin tins, spray the indentations and the rims around them with nonstick spray, or line the indentations with paper muffin cups. If using silicon muffin tins, spray as directed, then place them on a baking sheet.

2. Whisk the flour, sugar, cornmeal, baking soda, and fine salt in a medium bowl until well combined. Set aside.

3. In a large bowl, whisk the egg and sour cream until smooth. Whisk in the tequila, orange juice, oil, lime juice, and zest until well blended. Stir in the flour mixture with a wooden spoon until incorporated.

4. Fill the prepared tins three-quarters full. Use additional greased tins or small, oven-safe, greased ramekins for any leftover batter, or reserve the batter for a second bak-

ing. If desired, sprinkle 1/8 teaspoon coarse salt over each muffin top before baking. Bake for 20 minutes, or until the tops are lightly browned and cracked. A toothpick inserted into the center of one muffin should come out with a crumb or two attached.

5. Set the pan on a wire rack to cool for 10 minutes. Gently rock each muffin back and forth to release and remove it from the tin. Cool them for 5 minutes more on the rack before serving. If storing or freezing the muffins, cool them completely before sealing in an airtight container or in freezer-safe plastic bags. The muffins will stay fresh for up to 24 hours at room temperature or up to 1 month in the freezer.

Almond Margarita Muffins: *Omit the coarse salt. Sprinkle each muffin with 1 teaspoon sliced almonds before baking.*

Margarita Pumpkin Seed Muffins: *Add 3/4 cup toasted, shelled pumpkin seeds (or pepitas) with the flour.*

Mexican Chocolate Chip Margarita Muffins: *Add 1 teaspoon ground cinnamon with the flour. Stir in 1/3 cup mini semisweet chocolate chips and 1/3 cup toasted sliced almonds after the flour mixture.*

Sugar-Topped Margarita Muffins: *Omit the coarse salt. Sprinkle the muffins with 1/2 teaspoon coarse or colored sugar before baking (6 teaspoons total).*

Marmalade Muffins

Makes 12 muffins

Orange marmalade is a treat—a little sour, a little sweet, and very good with tea or coffee. In muffins, its strong flavor is mellowed considerably, yielding an extraordinarily subtle but still vivid taste. In our recipe, a little whole wheat flour further balances the taste, adding its own distinctive, earthy flavor. You can vary the basic recipe here by using other marmalades, like lemon or grapefruit, which are often available at specialty food stores.

Nonstick spray or paper muffin cups
2¹/₄ cups all-purpose flour
¹/₄ cup whole wheat flour or spelt flour
2 teaspoons baking soda
1 teaspoon baking powder
¹/₂ teaspoon salt
1 cup buttermilk (regular or low-fat)
³/₄ cup sugar
¹/₂ cup orange marmalade (see Note)
1 teaspoon grated lemon zest
2 large eggs, at room temperature
6 tablespoons (³/₄ stick) unsalted butter, melted and cooled
3 tablespoons Cointreau or other orange-flavored liqueur
1 teaspoon fresh lemon juice

1. Position the rack in the center of the oven and preheat the oven to 400°F. To prepare the muffin tins, spray the indentations and the rims around them with nonstick spray, or line the indentations with paper muffin cups. If using silicon muffin tins, spray as directed, then place them on a baking sheet.

2. Whisk the all-purpose flour, whole wheat flour, baking soda, baking powder, and salt in a large bowl until uniform. Set aside.

3. Place the buttermilk, sugar, marmalade, and lemon zest in a food processor fitted with the chopping blade or in a wide-canister blender; pulse or blend until the mixture is combined, then process until smooth, about 20 seconds. Scrape down the

sides of the bowl, then add the eggs, melted butter, Cointreau, and lemon juice. Process for an additional 20 seconds, or until smooth.

4. Pour the liquid mixture over the flour mixture; stir with a wooden spoon until the flour is incorporated. Do not overmix.

5. Fill the prepared tins three-quarters full. Use additional greased tins or individual, ovensafe, greased ramekins for any leftover batter, or reserve the batter for a second baking. Bake for 20 minutes, or until the muffins are pale brown with rounded, cracked tops. A toothpick inserted into the center of one muffin should come out with a crumb or two attached.

6. Set the pan on a wire rack to cool for 10 minutes. Gently rock each muffin back and forth to release and remove it from the tin. Cool them for 5 minutes more on the rack before serving. If storing or freezing the muffins, cool them completely before sealing in an airtight container or in freezer-safe plastic bags. The muffins will stay fresh for up to 24 hours at room temperature or up to 1 month in the freezer.

Note: *Although the best marmalade is made with whole, round slices of candied oranges, it makes for poor baking. Instead, look for marmalade that has tiny shreds or small pieces of rind in the jelly; this far cheaper variety will spread evenly throughout the batter.*

Brandied Marmalade Muffins: *Substitute brandy for the Cointreau.*

Chocolate Chip Marmalade Muffins: *Add 1/2 cup shaved semisweet chocolate or mini semisweet chocolate chips with the flour.*

Marmalade Streusel Muffins: *Top the muffins with Cinnamon Streusel Topping (page 224) before baking.*

Matzo Brei Muffins

Makes 12 muffins

Matzo is a flat cracker, served at Passover in Jewish homes when leavened bread is forbidden by religious law. Matzo Brei is made by soaking matzo in milk and eggs, then either scrambling the mixture or cooking it like a large pancake. These muffins will offer a third variation for matzo brei lovers of all generations.

$1/3$ cup canola or vegetable oil, plus additional for oiling the muffin tins

2 large egg yolks, at room temperature

$1^1/2$ cups milk (whole, low-fat, or nonfat)

3 matzo squares (each about 7 inches square)

4 large egg whites, at room temperature

$1/2$ teaspoon salt

$3/4$ cup maple syrup

1 teaspoon vanilla

$1^1/2$ cups matzo cake meal

1. Position the rack in the center of the oven and preheat the oven to 400°F. With a pastry brush or paper towel, lightly oil the muffin tins. If using silicon muffin tins, place them on a cookie sheet after oiling.

2. Whisk the egg yolks and milk in a large bowl until well blended. Crumble the matzos until they are in pieces the size of pocket change and stir them into the milk mixture until thoroughly coated. Set aside for 20 minutes, or until most of the liquid is absorbed.

3. Meanwhile, place the egg whites and salt in a large bowl and beat them with an electric mixer at high speed until soft peaks form, about 2 minutes, scraping down the sides of the bowl as necessary. Set aside.

4. Stir the remaining $1/3$ cup oil into the milk and matzo mixture, then stir in the maple syrup and vanilla extract until well combined. Finally, stir in the matzo cake meal.

5. Using a rubber spatula, fold one third of the beaten egg whites into the matzo mixture until no whites are visible. Then very gently fold in the remaining beaten egg whites until incorporated—there will still be white streaks in the batter.

6. Fill the prepared tins nearly to the top—these muffins will not rise very high. Bake for 25 minutes, or until the muffins are well browned and give some resistance when pressed. A toothpick inserted in the center of one muffin will come out with some wet crumbs attached.

7. Set the pan on a wire rack to cool for 10 minutes. Gently tip each muffin to one side to see if it's stuck. If one is, rock it back and forth to release it from the tin. Remove the muffins from the pan and cool them for 5 minutes more on the rack before serving. If storing, cool the muffins completely before sealing in an airtight container. The muffins will stay fresh for up to 24 hours at room temperature. We do not recommend freezing these muffins.

Apple Matzo Brei Muffins: *Whisk 1/2 teaspoon ground cinnamon with the eggs and milk. Add 3/4 cup chopped dried apple with the maple syrup.*

Apricot Nut Matzo Brei Muffins: *Add 1/3 cup chopped dried apricots and 1/3 cup chopped walnuts with the maple syrup.*

Date and Honey Matzo Brei Muffins: *Reduce the maple syrup to 1/2 cup. Add 1/4 cup honey and 2/3 cup chopped dates with the maple syrup.*

Matzo Brei Jam Muffins: *Fill the muffin tins halfway with batter, gently pressing it to the rims. Add 1 teaspoon jam, then top with the remaining batter to cover the jam.*

Matzo Brei Raisin Muffins: *Whisk 1/2 teaspoon ground cinnamon with the milk and eggs. Add 2/3 cup golden raisins with the maple syrup.*

Mexican Chocolate Muffins

Makes 12 muffins

These muffins bake up aromatic and luxurious, thanks to Mexican chocolate, a dark chocolate made with bits of cocoa nibs and ground cinnamon. Some brands also include ground almonds. For the best results, use Ibarra chocolate, sold in its unmistakable, round box.

Nonstick spray or paper muffin cups
Two 3.1-ounce Mexican chocolate bars, chopped
6 tablespoons ($^3/_4$ stick) unsalted butter
2$^1/_3$ cups all-purpose flour
2 teaspoons baking soda
$^1/_2$ teaspoon salt
2 large eggs, at room temperature
$^1/_3$ cup sugar
1 cup whole milk
$^1/_2$ teaspoon vanilla extract

1. Position the rack in the center of the oven and preheat the oven to 400°F. To prepare the muffin tins, spray the indentations and the rims around them with nonstick spray, or line the indentations with paper muffin cups. If using silicon muffin tins, spray as directed, then place them on a baking sheet.

2. Place the chocolate and butter in the top of a double boiler set over simmering water. If you don't have a double boiler, use a heatsafe bowl that fits snugly over a small pot of simmering water. Stir constantly until the chocolate and butter are half melted. Remove the top of the double boiler or the bowl from the pot; then continue stirring, away from the heat, until smooth. Cool for 10 minutes.

3. Meanwhile, whisk the flour, baking soda, and salt in a medium bowl until well blended. Set aside.

4. Once the chocolate mixture has cooled, whisk in the eggs one at a time, making sure the first is completely incorporated before adding the second. Whisk in the sugar until completely dissolved. Then whisk in the milk and vanilla until smooth, about 2 minutes.

5. Stir in the prepared flour mixture with a wooden spoon until incorporated. Do not overmix.

6. Fill the prepared tins three-quarters full. Use additional greased tins or small, oven-safe, greased ramekins for any leftover batter, or reserve the batter for a second baking. Bake for 20 minutes, or until the muffins have pale brown, smooth, rounded tops and a toothpick inserted in the center of one muffin comes out clean.

7. Set the pan on a wire rack to cool for 10 minutes. Gently rock each muffin back and forth to release and remove it from the tin. Cool them for 5 minutes more on the rack before serving. If storing or freezing the muffins, cool them completely before sealing in an airtight container or in freezer-safe plastic bags. The muffins will stay fresh for up to 24 hours at room temperature or up to 1 month in the freezer.

> **Mexican Chocolate Almond Muffins:** *Add 1 teaspoon almond extract and 1/2 cup toasted, sliced almonds with the vanilla.*
>
> **Mexican Chocolate Cinnamon Crunch Muffins:** *Top the muffins with Cinnamon Sugar Topping (page 225) before baking.*
>
> **Mexican Chocolate Chili Muffins:** *Add 1 tablespoon pure chili powder (that is, just ground chiles, with no added oregano or cumin) with the salt.*
>
> **Mexican Chocolate Papaya Muffins:** *Add 1/2 cup chopped dried papaya with the milk.*
>
> **Mexican Chocolate Pumpkin Seed Muffins:** *Add 1/2 cup toasted, shelled pumpkin seeds (pepitás) with the flour.*
>
> **Mexican Chocolate Sweet Peanut Muffins:** *Add 1/2 cup chopped honey-roasted peanuts with the milk.*

Nonfat Berry Muffins

Makes 12 muffins

Mashed bananas and nonfat yogurt are the secrets to keeping these muffins moist and light, but 2 cups of berries ensures that the flavor is bright and vivid.

Nonstick spray or paper muffin cups

3 egg whites, at room temperature

1$^{1}/_{2}$ cups plus 1 tablespoon all-purpose flour

$^{2}/_{3}$ cup sugar

$^{1}/_{2}$ cup yellow or white cornmeal

2 teaspoons baking powder

1 teaspoon baking soda

$^{1}/_{2}$ teaspoon salt

1 pint berries, hulled if necessary

2 large ripe bananas

$^{3}/_{4}$ cup nonfat yogurt

$^{1}/_{4}$ cup apple juice or water

1 teaspoon vanilla extract

1. Position the rack in the center of the oven and preheat the oven to 400°F. To prepare the muffin tins, spray the indentations and the rims around them with nonstick spray, or line the indentations with paper muffin cups. If using silicon muffin tins, spray as directed, then place them on a baking sheet.

2. Place the egg whites in a clean, dry, medium bowl; beat with an electric mixer at high speed until soft peaks form. Set aside.

3. In a second medium bowl, whisk the 1$^{1}/_{2}$ cups of flour, the sugar, cornmeal, baking powder, baking soda, and salt until uniform. In a small bowl, toss the berries with the remaining 1 tablespoon flour until well coated. Set both bowls aside.

4. Mash the bananas in a large bowl with a potato masher or a fork until smooth. Whisk in the yogurt, apple juice or water, and vanilla extract.

5. Stir in the flour mixture with a rubber spatula until moistened, then fold in the beaten egg whites, taking care not to press down and deflate the whites. Finally, once

there are just a few streaks of whites still in the batter, gently fold in the floured berries, taking care not to break them up.

6. Fill the muffin cups nearly to the top. Use additional greased tins or small, ovensafe, greased ramekins for any leftover batter, or reserve the batter for a second baking. Bake for 25 minutes, or until the muffins are brown with flat, cracked tops. A toothpick or cake tester, inserted in the middle of one muffin, will have a crumb or two attached, provided the berries don't gum it up.

7. Set the pan on a wire rack to cool for 10 minutes. Gently rock each muffin back and forth to release and remove it from the tin. Turn them upside down on the rack and cool the muffins for 5 minutes more. This stops the muffins from collapsing. Turn them over and serve, or let them stand on the wire rack until they are completely cooled before you seal them in an airtight container. They will stay fresh for up to 24 hours at room temperature. Because the berries remain whole, we do not recommend freezing these muffins.

Nonfat Berry Banana Chunk Muffins: *Reduce the berries to 1 cup. Toss 1 cup chopped dried bananas with the remaining berries and the flour.*

Nonfat Cinnamon Crunch Berry Muffins: *Top the muffins with Cinnamon Sugar Topping (page 225) before baking.*

Nonfat Double Berry Muffins: *Reduce the berries to 1 cup. Toss 1 cup dried cranberries, dried blueberries, dried cherries, or dried strawberries with the remaining fresh berries and the flour.*

Nonfat Spiced Berry Muffins: *Add 3/4 teaspoon ground cinnamon, 1/4 teaspoon grated nutmeg, 1/8 teaspoon ground cloves, and 1/8 teaspoon ground mace with the flour.*

Nonfat Corn Muffins

Makes 12 muffins

These dense muffins are not only nonfat, they're vegan—no eggs and no dairy whatsoever. But they still pack a wallop of corn flavor. Read labels carefully when buying your soy milk—use only nonfat; many brands contain high amounts of fat. And, for serving, don't forget to pick up some Concord grape jelly at the market as well.

Nonstick spray or paper muffin cups
1³/4 cups yellow or white cornmeal
1 cup all-purpose flour
1/4 cup sugar
1 tablespoon baking powder
1/2 teaspoon salt
One 14³/4-ounce can cream-style corn
1 cup nonfat soy milk

1. Position the rack in the center of the oven and preheat the oven to 375°F. To prepare the muffin tins, spray the indentations and the rims around them with nonstick spray, or line the indentations with paper muffin cups. If using silicon muffin tins, spray as directed, then place them on a baking sheet.

2. Whisk the cornmeal, flour, sugar, baking powder, and salt in a medium bowl until uniform. Set aside.

3. In a large bowl, whisk the cream-style corn and soy milk until well blended. Gently stir in the cornmeal mixture using a wooden spoon. Don't overmix—the batter should be quite grainy and even a little lumpy.

4. Fill the prepared tins three-quarters full. Use additional greased tins or small, oven-safe, greased ramekins for any leftover batter, or reserve the batter for a second baking. Bake for 20 minutes, or until the muffins have rounded, cracked tops, and a toothpick inserted in the center of one muffin comes out clean.

5. Set the pan on a wire rack to cool for 10 minutes. Gently rock each muffin back and forth to release it. Remove the muffins from the pan and cool for 5 minutes more on the rack before serving. If storing or freezing the muffins, cool them completely before sealing in an airtight container or in freezer-safe plastic bags. The muffins

will stay fresh for up to 24 hours at room temperature or up to 1 month in the freezer.

Nonfat Chili Corn Muffins: *Add 2 tablespoons chili powder with the flour. Add an additional tablespoon of nonfat soy milk.*

Nonfat Cilantro Corn Muffins: *Add 1/4 cup chopped fresh cilantro with the soy milk.*

Nonfat Cranberry Corn Muffins: *Add 3/4 cup dried cranberries with the soy milk.*

Nonfat Maple Corn Muffins: *Substitute maple sugar for the sugar.*

Oat Bran Muffins

Makes 12 muffins

Oat bran can give muffins a dry, grainy texture, so we've added walnut oil and buttermilk for body and flavor. When warm and velvety, these simple muffins are just waiting for jam or honey.

Nonstick spray or paper muffin cups
2 cups oat bran (see A Guide to Some Ingredients, page 11)
1 cup plus 2 tablespoons all-purpose flour
2$1/2$ teaspoons baking soda
$1/2$ teaspoon baking powder
$1/2$ teaspoon ground cinnamon
$1/2$ teaspoon salt
2 large eggs, at room temperature
$2/3$ cup packed light brown sugar
$3/4$ cup buttermilk (regular or low-fat)
$1/4$ cup walnut oil
1 teaspoon vanilla extract

1. Position the rack in the center of the oven and preheat the oven to 400°F. To prepare the muffin tins, spray the indentations and the rims around them with nonstick spray, or line the indentations with paper muffin cups. If using silicon muffin tins, spray as directed, then place them on a baking sheet.

2. Whisk the oat bran, flour, baking soda, baking powder, cinnamon, and salt in a medium bowl until well blended. Set aside.

3. In a large bowl, whisk the eggs until lightly beaten, then whisk in the brown sugar until thick and pale brown, about 2 minutes. Whisk in the buttermilk, oil, and vanilla until smooth. Stir in the prepared oat bran mixture until incorporated. The batter should be grainy with a few lumps—do not overmix.

4. Fill the prepared tins three-quarters full. Use additional greased tins or individual, ovensafe, greased ramekins for any leftover batter, or reserve the batter for a second baking. Bake for 20 minutes, or until the muffins are light browned with well

rounded tops and a toothpick inserted in the center of one muffin comes out with a crumb or two attached.

5. Set the pan on a wire rack to cool for 10 minutes. Gently rock each muffin back and forth to release and remove it from the tin. Cool them for 5 minutes more on the rack before serving. If storing or freezing the muffins, cool them completely before sealing in an airtight container or in freezer-safe plastic bags. The muffins will stay fresh for up to 24 hours at room temperature or up to 1 month in the freezer.

Apricot Pistachio Oat Bran Muffins: *Add 1/2 cup chopped dried apricots and 1/4 cup chopped, unsalted, shelled pistachios with the flour.*

Banana Oat Bran Muffins: *Add 3/4 cup chopped dried banana with the buttermilk.*

Lemon Glazed Oat Bran Muffins: *Top the cooled muffins with Lemon Drizzle (page 227).*

Oat Bran Date Nut Muffins: *Add 1/2 cup chopped, pitted dates and 1/4 cup chopped walnuts with the flour.*

Oat Bran Nut Crunch Muffins: *Top the muffins with Nut Crunch Topping (page 229) before baking.*

Plum Oat Bran Muffins: *Add 3/4 cup chopped dried plums with the flour.*

Prune Oat Bran Muffins: *Add 1/2 cup chopped, pitted prunes with the flour.*

Raisin Oat Bran Muffins: *Add 3/4 cup raisins with the flour.*

Oatmeal Muffins

Makes 12 muffins

Holiday egg casseroles may come and go, bacon may ride the tides of health fads, but oatmeal is one of those comforting breakfasts that simply endures. These muffins have the taste of oatmeal without the gumminess—as if we were finally able to get a bite of buttery toast and a spoonful of oatmeal in the same bite. The secret is to cut in the butter, as you would for a pastry dough. Don't wait for breakfast—bake these muffins the next time you have a craving for oatmeal cookies but want something that takes less time.

Nonstick spray or paper muffin cups

$1^1/2$ cups rolled oats (do not use quick-cooking oats)

$1^1/4$ cups all-purpose flour

2 teaspoons baking soda

1 teaspoon baking powder

$1/2$ teaspoon ground cinnamon

$1/2$ teaspoon salt

6 tablespoons ($3/4$ stick) cold, unsalted butter, cut into small chunks

2 large eggs, at room temperature

$1/2$ cup packed light brown sugar

1 cup buttermilk (regular or low-fat)

2 teaspoons vanilla extract

1 cup raisins

1. Position the rack in the center of the oven and preheat the oven to 400°F. To prepare the muffin tins, spray the indentations and the rims around them with nonstick spray, or line the indentations with paper muffin cups. If using silicon muffin tins, spray as directed, then place them on a baking sheet.

2. Whisk the oats, flour, baking soda, baking powder, cinnamon, and salt in a medium bowl until well blended. Cut in the butter, using a pastry cutter or two forks, until the mixture resembles coarse meal.

3. In a large bowl, whisk the eggs until lightly beaten. Add the brown sugar; continue whisking until the mixture is thick and pale yellow, about 2 minutes. Whisk in the

buttermilk and vanilla until smooth. Pour in the raisins, stir until combined, then stir in the prepared oat mixture until moistened.

4. Fill the prepared tins three-quarters full. Use additional greased tins or individual, ovensafe, greased ramekins for any leftover batter, or reserve the batter for a second baking. Bake for 20 minutes, or until the muffins are lightly browned with rounded tops and a toothpick inserted in the center of one muffin comes out clean.

5. Set the pan on a wire rack to cool for 10 minutes. Gently rock each muffin back and forth to release and remove it from the tin. Cool them for 5 minutes more on the rack before serving. If storing or freezing the muffins, cool them completely before sealing in an airtight container or in freezer-safe plastic bags. The muffins will stay fresh for up to 24 hours at room temperature or up to 1 month in the freezer.

> **Oatmeal Apricot Muffins:** *Substitute 1 cup chopped dried apricots for the raisins.*
>
> **Oatmeal Peanut Butter Muffins:** *Fill the tins one-third full, gently spreading the batter to the rims. Place 1 teaspoon smooth or crunchy peanut butter on top of the batter in each tin, then divide the remaining batter equally among the tins until they are three-quarters full, covering the peanut butter.*
>
> **Oatmeal Rainbow Muffins:** *Substitute 1 cup mini M&M candies for the raisins.*
>
> **Raisin Walnut Oatmeal Muffins:** *Reduce the raisins to 1/2 cup. Add 1/2 cup chopped walnuts with the remaining raisins.*
>
> **Vanilla Glazed Oatmeal Cranberry Muffins:** *Substitute dried cranberries for the raisins. Coat the cooled muffins with Vanilla Dip (page 231).*

Olive Oil Muffins

Makes 12 muffins

Olive oil cakes have a long history in Italian cooking. They're usually made with semolina for texture, a coarsely ground flour made from durum wheat; it can be hard to find, so white or yellow cornmeal can give a similar, if slightly crunchier, texture to the muffins. In any case, olive oil cakes are always flavored with a cook's most highly prized olive oil. To re-create that taste in these muffins, use extra virgin olive oil, preferably one that's labeled "first cold pressed," an oil produced from fresh olives without any heat and so without any of the olive flavor being volatilized or steamed off. Try these muffins with eggs, a frittata, or even pasta. They're also terrific with cocktails before an Italian dinner—warm, split open, and topped with olive tapenade or a little sour cream and caviar.

Nonstick spray or paper muffin cups
1¹/2 cups all-purpose flour
¹/2 cup semolina or cornmeal (preferably white)
¹/2 cup sugar
2 teaspoons baking powder
1 teaspoon baking soda
1 teaspoon salt
2 large eggs, at room temperature
³/4 cup milk (whole, low-fat, or nonfat)
¹/4 cup Marsala wine (see Note)
³/4 cup extra virgin olive oil
1¹/2 teaspoons grated lemon zest

1. Position the rack in the center of the oven and preheat the oven to 400°F. To prepare the muffin tins, spray the indentations and the rims around them with nonstick spray, or line the indentations with paper muffin cups. If using silicon muffin tins, spray as directed, then place them on a baking sheet.

2. Whisk the flour, semolina or cornmeal, sugar, baking powder, baking soda, and salt until uniform. Set aside.

3. In a large bowl, whisk the eggs, milk, and Marsala until smooth; whisk in the olive oil and lemon zest. Stir in the prepared flour mixture with a wooden spoon until moistened.

4. Fill the prepared tins three-quarters full. Use additional greased tins or individual, ovensafe, greased ramekins for any leftover batter, or reserve the batter for a second baking. Bake for 20 minutes, or until the muffins are lightly browned with rounded, lightly cracked tops. A toothpick inserted into the center of one muffin should come out with a few moist crumbs attached.

5. Set the pan on a wire rack to cool for 10 minutes. Gently rock each muffin back and forth to release and remove it from the tin. Cool them for 5 minutes more on the rack before serving. If storing or freezing the muffins, cool them completely before sealing in an airtight container or in freezer-safe plastic bags. The muffins will stay fresh for up to 24 hours at room temperature or up to 1 month in the freezer.

Note: *This aged, fortified Sicilian wine lends a perfume-like aroma to the muffins. In a pinch, you can substitute Madeira or even sherry, although the taste will not be as heady.*

> **Herbed Goat Cheese Olive Oil Muffins:** *Crumble 1/2 cup herbed goat cheese (about 2 ounces) into the batter just before adding the prepared flour mixture.*
>
> **Olive Rosemary Muffins:** *Mix 1/2 cup chopped pitted green or black olives and 2 teaspoons chopped fresh rosemary into the batter just before adding the prepared flour mixture.*
>
> **Pesto Muffins:** *Mix 1/4 cup finely chopped fresh basil, 1 clove minced fresh garlic, and 2 tablespoons chopped pine nuts into the batter just before adding the prepared flour mixture.*
>
> **Sun-Dried Tomato Olive Oil Muffins:** *Mix 1/3 cup marinated sun-dried tomatoes, drained and chopped, into the batter just before adding the prepared flour mixture.*

Orange Muffins

Makes 12 muffins

In Shakespeare's world, you didn't turn green with envy—you turned orange. A rarity back then, oranges were considered a dangerous fruit, railed against by preachers and physicians: they were too sweet, too sour, too everything. They could set you in a tizzy, throwing your body's humors out of whack, the same way envy could. We make no such claim, but do know that that very confluence of flavors in an orange—sweet, sour, acidic, and a little bitter—makes for dynamic muffins. Orange oil, offered here as an option, is simply the essential oil found in the peel and is available in most gourmet stores and many supermarkets in the spice or baking supply section.

Nonstick spray or paper muffin cups
2¼ cups all-purpose flour
¾ cup sugar
2 teaspoons baking soda
½ teaspoon salt
1 large egg, at room temperature
½ cup yogurt (regular, low-fat, or nonfat)
6 tablespoons (¾ stick) unsalted butter, melted and cooled
1 tablespoon finely grated orange zest
¾ cup orange juice (see Note)
¼ cup milk (whole, low-fat, or nonfat)
¼ teaspoon orange oil (optional)

1. Position the rack in the center of the oven and preheat the oven to 400°F. To prepare the muffin tins, spray the indentations and the rims around them with nonstick spray, or line the indentations with paper muffin cups. If using silicon muffin tins, spray as directed, then place them on a baking sheet.

2. Whisk the flour, sugar, baking soda, and salt in a medium bowl until uniform. Set aside.

3. In a large bowl, whisk the egg and yogurt until smooth, then whisk in the melted butter and orange zest. Once incorporated, whisk in the orange juice, milk, and orange oil, if using. Finally, stir in the prepared flour mixture with a wooden spoon until moistened.

4. Fill the prepared tins three-quarters full. Use additional greased tins or individual, ovensafe, greased ramekins for any leftover batter, or reserve the batter for a second baking. Bake for 20 minutes, or until the tops are rounded and lightly brown. A toothpick inserted in the center of one muffin should come out with a few moist crumbs attached.

5. Set the pan on a wire rack to cool for 10 minutes. Gently rock each muffin back and forth to release and remove it from the tin. Cool them for 5 minutes more on the rack before serving. If storing or freezing the muffins, cool them completely before sealing in an airtight container or in freezer-safe plastic bags. The muffins will stay fresh for up to 24 hours at room temperature or up to 1 month in the freezer.

Note: *For the best flavor, squeeze your own orange juice. Use oranges at room temperature and roll them along the counter, pressing down with your palm, before slicing them open and juicing them.*

> **Blood Red Orange Muffins:** *Substitute blood orange juice and zest for the orange juice and zest. Whisk in 6 drops red food coloring, if desired, with the yogurt.*
>
> **Chocolate Chip Orange Muffins:** *Add 3/4 cup miniature milk chocolate chips with the flour.*
>
> **Minty Orange Muffins:** *Add 2 tablespoons chopped fresh mint with the orange zest.*
>
> **Moroccan Orange Muffins:** *Add 1 teaspoon ground cinnamon, 1/2 teaspoon ground cumin, 1/2 teaspoon ground mustard, and 1/8 teaspoon crumbled saffron with the flour.*
>
> **Orange Walnut Crunch Muffins:** *Add 2/3 cup toasted chopped walnuts with the flour. Top the muffins with Cinnamon Streusel Topping (page 224) before baking.*
>
> **Provençal Savory Muffins:** *Add 2 tablespoons chopped fresh rosemary with the yogurt. Reduce the butter to 3 tablespoons, and add 3 tablespoons olive oil with the remaining butter.*
>
> **Three Citrus Muffins:** *Substitute grapefruit juice for the orange juice. Substitute grapefruit or lemon zest for the orange zest. Do not use any orange oil.*

Parmesan Muffins

Makes 12 muffins

Parmesan bread has become an American bakery staple—a dense bread laced with the famous cheese from Italy. Our version is something of a cross between a savory muffin and a biscuit—it's a little denser than some of the other muffins, and thus the perfect thing to serve with dinner instead of bread.

Nonstick spray or paper muffin cups
2 cups all-purpose flour
$3/4$ cup grated Parmigiano-Reggiano (about 4 ounces)
$1/4$ cup sugar
1 tablespoon baking powder
1 teaspoon sweet paprika
$1/2$ teaspoon salt
1 large egg, at room temperature
$1/2$ cup sour cream (regular, low-fat, or nonfat)
$2/3$ cup milk (whole, low-fat, or nonfat)
$1/2$ cup canola or vegetable oil

1. Position the rack in the center of the oven and preheat the oven to 400°F. To prepare the muffin tins, spray the indentations and the rims around them with nonstick spray, or line the indentations with paper muffin cups. If using silicon muffin tins, spray as directed, then place them on a baking sheet.

2. Whisk the flour, $1/2$ cup of the grated cheese, the sugar, baking powder, paprika, and salt in a medium bowl until well combined. Set aside.

3. In a large bowl, whisk the egg and sour cream until smooth, then whisk in the milk and oil. Use a wooden spoon to stir in the prepared flour mixture until moistened.

4. Fill the prepared tins three-quarters full. Use additional greased tins or individual, ovensafe, greased ramekins for any leftover batter, or reserve the batter for a second baking. Sprinkle 1 teaspoon of the remaining grated cheese over the top of each muffin. Bake for 20 minutes, or until the muffins are pale brown with rounded, cracked tops. A toothpick inserted into the center of one muffin should come out clean.

5. Set the pan on a wire rack to cool for 10 minutes. Gently rock each muffin back and forth to release and remove it from the tin. Cool them for 5 minutes more on the rack before serving. If storing or freezing the muffins, cool them completely before sealing in an airtight container or in freezer-safe plastic bags. The muffins will stay fresh for up to 24 hours at room temperature or up to 1 month in the freezer.

Fiery Parmesan Muffins: *Substitute hot Hungarian paprika for the sweet paprika.*

Green Onion Parmesan Muffins: *Thinly slice 3 large green onions and sauté in a small skillet with 1 tablespoon olive oil over medium heat for 1 minute or until softened. Add the cooked green onions to the batter with the milk.*

Mustard Dill Parmesan Muffins: *Add 1 tablespoon Dijon mustard and 2 tablespoons chopped fresh dill with the milk.*

Parmesan Cornmeal Muffins: *Reduce the flour to 1 1/4 cups; whisk in 3/4 cup yellow cornmeal with the remaining flour.*

Parmesan Olive Oil Muffins: *Substitute olive oil for the canola oil.*

Pimiento Parmesan Muffins: *Add one 6-ounce jar chopped pimientos, drained, with the milk.*

Roasted Garlic Parmesan Muffins: *Roast a garlic head as indicated on page 188. Cool, then squeeze out the softened cloves and whisk them in with the oil, breaking up any bits of garlic as you whisk.*

Peach Muffins

Makes 12 muffins

The global food distribution network has ensured we will have lots of peaches, but since they're picked green and shipped over thousands of miles, they're often mealy and tasteless. A shame, yes—but not the death knell for peach muffins, since the muffins can best be made with frozen peaches, which are often packaged when ripe, even overripe, ensuring better muffins every time.

Nonstick spray or paper muffin cups
1³/4 cups all-purpose flour
1/4 cup yellow cornmeal
2¹/2 teaspoons baking soda
1/2 teaspoon baking powder
1/2 teaspoon salt
One 1-pound bag frozen peach slices, thawed in the bag
2 large eggs, at room temperature
1/2 cup sugar
2 teaspoons vanilla extract
6 tablespoons (³/4 stick) unsalted butter, melted and cooled
1/3 cup buttermilk (regular or low-fat)
1/3 cup yogurt (regular, low-fat, or nonfat)

1. Position the rack in the center of the oven and preheat the oven to 400°F. To prepare the muffin tins, spray the indentations and the rims around them with nonstick spray, or line the indentations with paper muffin cups. If using silicon muffin tins, spray as directed, then place them on a baking sheet.

2. In a medium bowl, whisk the flour, cornmeal, baking soda, baking powder, and salt until well combined. Set aside.

3. Drain the peaches, reserving the liquid. Place 2 cups of the peach slices along with the reserved liquid in a food processor fitted with the chopping blade or a wide-canister blender. Add the eggs, sugar, and vanilla. Process or blend for 1 minute or until smooth, scraping down the sides of the bowl as necessary. Transfer this purée to a large bowl.

4. Roughly chop the remaining peach slices and stir them into the purée along with the melted butter, buttermilk, and yogurt. Stir until well blended, then quickly stir in the prepared flour mixture until moistened.

5. Fill the prepared tins three-quarters full. Use additional greased tins or individual, ovensafe, greased ramekins for any leftover batter, or reserve the batter for a second baking. Bake for 23 minutes, or until the muffins tops are lightly browned and a toothpick inserted in the center of one muffin comes out with a few moist crumbs attached.

6. Set the pan on a wire rack to cool for 10 minutes. Gently rock each muffin back and forth to release and remove it from the tin. Cool them for 5 minutes more on the rack before serving. If storing or freezing the muffins, cool them completely before sealing in an airtight container or in freezer-safe plastic bags. The muffins will stay fresh for up to 24 hours at room temperature or up to 1 month in the freezer.

Peach Almond Muffins: *Reduce the vanilla to 1 teaspoon. Add 1/2 teaspoon almond extract with the remaining vanilla. Stir in 1/2 cup toasted, sliced almonds with the chopped peach slices.*

Peach Cinnamon Crunch Muffins: *Top the muffins with Cinnamon Sugar Topping (page 225) before baking.*

Peach Coconut Muffins: *Add 2/3 cup shredded sweetened coconut with the chopped peach slices.*

Peach Melba Muffins: *Increase the cornmeal to 1/3 cup. Gently fold 1 cup raspberries into the batter with the flour mixture.*

Peach Pie Muffins: *Add 1 teaspoon ground cinnamon, 1/2 teaspoon grated nutmeg, and 1/4 teaspoon ground cloves with the flour.*

Peach Streusel Muffins: *Top the muffins with Cinnamon Streusel Topping (page 224) before baking.*

Peach Sundae Muffins: *Top each muffin with a maraschino cherry (minus the stem) before baking.*

Vanilla Peach Glazed Muffins: *Coat the cooled muffins with Vanilla Dip (page 231).*

Peanut Butter Muffins

Makes 12 muffins

Not sweet enough to be cupcakes, these muffins taste more like warm, freshly-baked peanut butter cookies. Serve them with plenty of jelly, Marshmallow Fluff, or honey. If you're an Elvis fan, don't overlook the variations, especially the Peanut Butter Bacon Banana Muffins.

Nonstick spray or paper muffin cups
1³/4 cups all-purpose flour
1 tablespoon baking powder
1/2 teaspoon salt
1 large egg, at room temperature
1/2 cup packed light brown sugar
2/3 cup smooth peanut butter
1¹/4 cups milk (whole, low-fat, or nonfat)
5 tablespoons unsalted butter, melted and cooled
1 teaspoon vanilla extract

1. Position the rack in the center of the oven and preheat the oven to 400°F. To prepare the muffin tins, spray the indentations and the rims around them with nonstick spray, or line the indentations with paper muffin cups. If using silicon muffin tins, spray as directed, then place them on a baking sheet.

2. Whisk the flour, baking powder, and salt in a small bowl until well combined. Set aside.

3. In a large bowl, whisk the eggs until lightly beaten. Whisk in the brown sugar and continue whisking until thick, smooth, and pale brown, about 2 minutes. Whisk in the peanut butter until smooth, then stir in the milk, melted butter, and vanilla. Use a wooden spoon to stir in the flour mixture, until incorporated. The batter is quite thick; be careful not to overmix.

4. Fill the prepared tins three-quarters full. Use additional greased tins or individual, ovensafe, greased ramekins for any leftover batter, or reserve the batter for a second baking. Bake for 20 minutes, or until the muffins are lightly browned with rounded

tops. A toothpick inserted into the center of one muffin should come out with a crumb or two attached.

5. Set the pan on a wire rack to cool for 10 minutes. Gently rock each muffin back and forth to release and remove it from the tin. Cool them for 5 minutes more on the rack before serving. If storing or freezing the muffins, cool them completely before sealing in an airtight container or in freezer-safe plastic bags. The muffins will stay fresh for up to 2 days at room temperature or up to 3 months in the freezer.

> **Crunchy Peanut Butter Muffins:** *Mix in 1/2 cup chopped, unsalted, roasted peanuts with the milk.*
>
> **Peanut Butter and Jelly Muffins:** *Fill the muffin tins one-third full, gently spreading the batter to the rims. Place 1 teaspoon jelly on top of the batter in each tin, then divide the remaining batter equally among the tins, covering the jelly completely.*
>
> **Peanut Butter Bacon Banana Muffins:** *Fry three strips of bacon until crisp. Drain and crumble them into the batter with the milk. Also add 1/4 cup chopped dried banana with the milk. (Call them Elvis muffins!)*
>
> **Peanut Butter Chocolate Chip Muffins:** *Add 3/4 cup milk chocolate chips with the flour.*
>
> **Peanut Butter Cinnamon Crunch Muffins:** *Top the muffins with Cinnamon Sugar Topping (page 225) before baking.*
>
> **Sweet Peanut Butter Chunk Muffins:** *Add 3/4 cup peanut butter chips with the flour.*
>
> **White Chocolate Chip Peanut Butter Muffins:** *Add 3/4 cup white chocolate chips with the flour.*

Pear Muffins

Makes 12 muffins

To choose the best pears, there's only one rule, the same for any fruit: if they don't smell like anything, they probably won't taste like anything. For these muffins, choose firm pears, ones that are brightly fragrant. You can ripen them on the counter in a paper bag overnight, but make sure they don't get too soft, since you'll need to grate them into the batter.

Nonstick spray or paper muffin cups
3 firm, medium pears (about 8 ounces each)
1 cup packed light brown sugar
2 cups all-purpose flour
2 teaspoons baking powder
1 teaspoon baking soda
1/2 teaspoon salt
1/4 teaspoon ground ginger
1 large egg, lightly beaten, at room temperature
1/2 cup plain yogurt (regular, low-fat, or nonfat)
1/4 cup canola or vegetable oil
1/4 cup pear nectar
1 teaspoon grated lemon zest

1. Position the rack in the center of the oven and preheat the oven to 400°F. To prepare the muffin tins, spray the indentations and the rims around them with nonstick spray, or line the indentations with paper muffin cups. If using silicon muffin tins, spray as directed, then place them on a baking sheet.

2. Peel and core the pears. Shred them into a large bowl, using the large holes of a box grater. Stir in the brown sugar, toss well, and set aside for 30 minutes.

3. Whisk the flour, baking powder, baking soda, salt, and ground ginger in a medium bowl until uniform. Set aside.

4. Using a wooden spoon, stir the egg into the shredded pears, then stir in the yogurt, oil, pear nectar, and lemon zest until smooth. Stir in the prepared flour mixture just until incorporated.

5. Fill the prepared tins three-quarters full. Use additional greased tins or individual, ovensafe, greased ramekins for any leftover batter, or reserve the batter for a second baking. Bake for 23 minutes, or until the muffins are light brown with rounded tops. A toothpick inserted into the center of one muffin should come out with a crumb or two attached.

6. Set the pan on a wire rack to cool for 10 minutes. Gently rock each muffin back and forth to release and remove it from the tin. Cool them for 5 minutes more on the rack before serving. If storing or freezing the muffins, cool them completely before sealing in an airtight container or in freezer-safe plastic bags. The muffins will stay fresh for up to 2 days at room temperature or up to 2 months in the freezer.

> **Lemon Glazed Pear Muffins:** *Top the cooled muffins with Lemon Drizzle (page 227).*
>
> **Pear Cranberry Muffins:** *Use only two pears. Add 1 cup chopped fresh cranberries with the egg.*
>
> **Pear Oat Crunch Muffins:** *Top the muffins with Oat Crunch Topping (page 230) before baking.*
>
> **Pear Parmesan Muffins:** *Add 1/2 cup grated Parmigiano-Reggiano with the egg.*
>
> **Pear Raisin Muffins:** *Add 3/4 cup golden raisins with the yogurt.*
>
> **Pear Walnut Muffins:** *Substitute walnut oil for the canola oil. Add 3/4 cup chopped toasted walnuts with the yogurt.*

Pecan Muffins

Makes 12 muffins

Don't let the maple syrup and brown sugar fool you. The stunning flavor of toasted pecans infuses these muffins without ever making them taste like brittle or candy crunch.

Nonstick spray or paper muffin cups
2 cups chopped pecan pieces
1^1/2 cups all-purpose flour
2 teaspoons baking soda
^{1}/2 teaspoon baking powder
^{1}/2 teaspoon salt
2 large eggs, at room temperature
^{1}/4 cup packed dark brown sugar
^{1}/4 cup maple syrup
^{1}/2 cup buttermilk (regular or low-fat)
4 tablespoons (^{1}/2 stick) unsalted butter, melted and cooled
1 teaspoon vanilla extract

1. Position the rack in the center of the oven and preheat the oven to 400°F. To prepare the muffin tins, spray the indentations and the rims around them with nonstick spray, or line the indentations with paper muffin cups. If using silicon muffin tins, spray as directed, then place them on a baking sheet.

2. Spread the pecans on a baking sheet and place them in the oven for about 7 minutes, stirring frequently, until golden brown and fragrant. Remove from the oven and cool for 10 minutes. Maintain the oven temperature.

3. Whisk the flour, baking soda, baking powder, and salt in a medium bowl until uniform. Set aside.

4. In a large bowl, whisk the eggs until lightly beaten, then whisk in the brown sugar and maple syrup until thick and pale brown, about 2 minutes. Whisk in the buttermilk, melted butter, and vanilla until smooth. Chop the cooled nuts and stir them into the batter, then stir in the prepared flour mixture until incorporated. Do not overmix.

5. Fill the prepared tins three-quarters full. Use additional greased tins or individual, ovensafe, greased ramekins for any leftover batter, or reserve the batter for a second baking. Bake for 20 minutes, or until the tops are rounded and lightly browned and a toothpick inserted in the center of one muffin comes out with a few crumbs attached.

6. Set the pan on a wire rack to cool for 10 minutes. Gently rock each muffin back and forth to release and remove it from the tin. Cool them for 5 minutes more on the rack before serving. If storing or freezing the muffins, cool them completely before sealing in an airtight container or in freezer-safe plastic bags. The muffins will stay fresh for up to 24 hours at room temperature or up to 1 month in the freezer.

> **Chocolate Crunch Pecan Muffins:** *Top the muffins with Chocolate Crunch Topping (page 222) before baking.*
>
> **Cinnamon Pecan Crunch Muffins:** *Top the muffins with Cinnamon Sugar Topping (page 225) before baking.*
>
> **Pecan Cherry Muffins:** *Add 2/3 cup dried cherries with the chopped pecans.*
>
> **Pecan Cocoa Nib Muffins:** *Add 1/2 cup cocoa nibs with the chopped pecans.*
>
> **Pecan Cranberry Muffins:** *Add 2/3 cup dried cranberries with the chopped pecans.*
>
> **Pecan Crumb Muffins:** *Top the muffins with Crumb Topping (page 226) before baking.*
>
> **Pecan Oat Muffins:** *Substitute 1/2 cup oat flour for 1/2 cup of the all-purpose flour. Top each muffin with 1 1/2 teaspoons rolled oats (do not use quick-cooking oats) before baking.*
>
> **Pecan Peanut Butter Muffins:** *Add 2/3 cup peanut butter chips with the chopped pecans.*
>
> **Pecan Raisin Muffins:** *Add 2/3 cup raisins with the chopped pecans.*
>
> **Vanilla Glazed Pecan Muffins:** *Coat the cooled muffins with Vanilla Dip (page 231).*

Piña Colada Muffins

Makes 12 muffins

A piña colada was one of those cocktails that came into vogue in the '70s, thanks to the disco craze, and has stayed on as a staple—at least at tiki bars and retro cocktail parties. The combination of rum, pineapple, and coconut is irresistible in the cocktail and in these dessert muffins, sweetened with canned cream of coconut.

Nonstick spray or paper muffin cups
2^1/3 cups all-purpose flour
2 teaspoons baking soda
1 teaspoon baking powder
^{1}/2 teaspoon salt
One 12-ounce can cream of coconut (see page 13)
One 8-ounce can crushed pineapple in juice, drained
^{1}/4 cup white or gold rum (do not use dark rum)
1 large egg, at room temperature

1. Position the rack in the center of the oven and preheat the oven to 400°F. To prepare the muffin tins, spray the indentations and the rims around them with nonstick spray, or line the indentations with paper muffin cups. If using silicon muffin tins, spray as directed, then place them on a baking sheet.

2. Whisk the flour, baking soda, baking powder, and salt in a medium bowl until uniform. Set aside.

3. In a large bowl, whisk the cream of coconut, pineapple, rum, and egg until well blended. Stir in the flour mixture until moistened.

4. Fill the prepared tins three-quarters full. Use additional greased tins or individual, ovensafe, greased ramekins for any leftover batter, or reserve the batter for a second baking. Bake for 23 minutes, or until the muffins are well browned and a toothpick inserted in the center of one muffin comes out with a few moist crumbs attached.

5. Set the pan on a wire rack to cool for 10 minutes. Gently tip each muffin to one side to make sure it isn't stuck. If one is, gently rock it back and forth to release it from the tin. Remove the muffins and cool for 5 minutes more on the rack before serving. If storing or freezing the muffins, cool them completely before sealing in an air-

tight container or in freezer-safe plastic bags. The muffins will stay fresh for up to 2 days at room temperature or up to 2 months in the freezer.

Apricot Piña Colada Muffins: *Substitute 1/4 cup apricot brandy for the rum.*

Cinnamon Crunch Piña Colada Muffins: *Top the muffins with Cinnamon Sugar Topping (page 225) before baking.*

Double Coconut Piña Colada Muffins: *Substitute coconut rum for the white or gold rum.*

Lemon Glazed Piña Colada Muffins: *Top the cooled muffins with Lemon Drizzle (page 227).*

Nut Crunch Piña Colada Muffins: *Top the muffins with Nut Crunch Topping (page 229) before baking.*

Vanilla Almond Piña Colada Muffins: *Add 2 teaspoons vanilla extract with the rum. Sprinkle each muffin with 2 teaspoons sliced almonds before baking.*

Vanilla Glazed Piña Colada Muffins: *Coat the cooled muffins with Vanilla Dip (page 231).*

Virgin Piña Colada Muffins: *Omit the rum. Add 1 teaspoon rum extract and 1/4 cup pineapple juice (reserved from the canned pineapple) with the cream of coconut.*

Pine Nut Muffins

Makes 12 muffins

Harvested from the cones of certain pine trees, pine nuts are quintessentially Mediterranean. They're aromatic like almonds but have the distinct taste of pine resin, light and heady. They can go rancid quite quickly, so store them tightly sealed in your freezer until you're ready to use them. In these muffins, soft ricotta cheese is added for richness and a light, tangy taste, typical of some Italian pastries.

Nonstick spray or paper muffin cups
3/4 cup pine nuts
2 cups all-purpose flour
2/3 cup sugar
1 tablespoon baking powder
1 teaspoon salt
2 large eggs, at room temperature
3/4 cup ricotta cheese (whole-milk or low-fat, but not nonfat)
3/4 cup milk (whole, low-fat, or nonfat)
1/2 cup canola or vegetable oil
1 teaspoon vanilla extract

1. Position the rack in the center of the oven and preheat the oven to 400°F. To prepare the muffin tins, spray the indentations and the rims around them with nonstick spray, or line the indentations with paper muffin cups. If using silicon muffin tins, spray as directed, then place them on a baking sheet.

2. Place the pine nuts on a baking sheet and bake for 6 minutes, stirring occasionally, until lightly brown and fragrant. Transfer the nuts to a large plate and cool for 10 minutes. Maintain the oven's temperature.

3. Pour 1/3 cup of the toasted nuts into a food processor, a mini food processor, or a blender; pulse 5 or 6 times until the nuts are finely ground. Be careful not to grind them into a paste. Transfer the ground nuts to a medium bowl. Stir in the flour, sugar, baking powder, salt, and the remaining pine nuts until well combined.

4. Whisk the eggs and ricotta in a large bowl, then whisk in the milk, oil, and vanilla until smooth. Use a wooden spoon to stir in the prepared flour mixture until

moistened. Make sure the pine nuts are evenly distributed in the batter, but do not overmix.

5. Fill the prepared tins three-quarters full. Use additional greased tins or individual, ovensafe, greased ramekins for any leftover batter, or reserve the batter for a second baking. Bake for 22 minutes, or until the muffins are pale brown with rounded, cracked tops. A toothpick inserted into the center of one muffin should come out with a few moist crumbs attached.

6. Set the pan on a wire rack to cool for 10 minutes. Gently rock each muffin back and forth to release and remove it from the tin. Cool them for 5 minutes more on the rack before serving. If storing or freezing the muffins, cool them completely before sealing in an airtight container or in freezer-safe plastic bags. The muffins will stay fresh for up to 24 hours at room temperature or up to 1 month in the freezer.

> **Anise Raisin Pine Nut Muffins:** *Add 1/3 cup raisins and 2 teaspoons anise seeds with the flour.*
>
> **Lemon Pine Nut Muffins:** *Reduce the milk by 2 teaspoons. Add 2 teaspoons grated fresh lemon zest and 2 teaspoons fresh lemon juice with the oil.*
>
> **Maple Pine Nut Muffins:** *Sprinkle each muffin with 1 teaspoon maple sugar before baking.*
>
> **Tropical Pine Nut Muffins:** *Add 3 tablespoons chopped dried pineapple and 3 tablespoons sweetened shredded coconut with the oil.*

Pineapple Upside-Down Muffins

Makes 12 muffins

The bottoms of these muffins are rich and gooey—with sweet pineapple and a baked-on caramel syrup. Remove them from the tins and serve them upside down so as not to lose any of the pineapple bottoms. Make sure your tins are well greased. These muffins cannot be made in paper muffin cups.

Nonstick spray

3 tablespoons packed light brown sugar

8 tablespoons (1 stick) unsalted butter, melted and cooled

One 8-ounce can crushed pineapple in heavy syrup, drained

2 cups plus 2 tablespoons all-purpose flour

$1/2$ cup granulated sugar

2 teaspoons baking powder

1 teaspoon baking soda

$1/2$ teaspoon salt

2 large eggs, at room temperature

$3/4$ cup buttermilk (regular or low-fat)

$1/4$ teaspoon almond extract

1. Position the rack in the center of the oven and preheat the oven to 375°F. To prepare the muffin tins, spray the indentations and the rims around them with nonstick spray. If using silicon muffin tins, place the tins on a baking sheet after spraying.

2. In a small bowl, mix the brown sugar and 2 tablespoons of the melted butter until well combined. Divide this mixture evenly among the 12 muffin tins, placing about 1 teaspoon in the bottom of each. Top the butter mixture in each tin with 1 teaspoon of crushed pineapple. Set aside.

3. Whisk the flour, granulated sugar, baking powder, baking soda, and salt until uniform. Set aside.

4. In large bowl, whisk the eggs until frothy. Whisk in the buttermilk, the almond extract, the remaining 6 tablespoons melted butter, and the remaining crushed pineapple. Gently stir in the prepared flour mixture with a wooden spoon until moistened.

5. Taking care not to disturb the sugar and pineapple in the bottom of the tins, fill them three-quarters full with batter. Use additional greased tins or individual ovensafe, greased ramekins for any leftover batter, or reserve the batter for a second baking. Bake for 22 minutes, or until the muffins are lightly browned with rounded tops. A toothpick inserted into the center of one muffin should come out with a few moist crumbs attached.

6. Set the pan on a wire rack to cool for 15 minutes. Gently tip each muffin to one side, taking care to keep the pineapple bottom attached. If it comes loose, simply scrape it out and gently press it back onto the muffin top once the muffin has been removed from the tin. Remove all the muffins; serve them upside down. Cool completely before sealing them in an airtight container, where they will stay fresh for up to 2 days. These muffins do not freeze well.

> **Hawaiian Nut Pineapple Upside-Down Muffins:** *Add 1/2 cup chopped macadamia nuts with the buttermilk.*
>
> **Pineapple Rum Upside-Down Muffins:** *Drizzle 1 teaspoon white or gold rum over the bottoms of each warm muffin after they have been removed from the tins.*
>
> **Pineapple Upside-Down Fruit Cake Muffins:** *Place 1 glacéed cherry and 1 pecan half in the bottom of each muffin tin along with the crushed pineapple and brown sugar mixture.*

Pizza Muffins

Makes 12 muffins

All sorts of pizza toppings are mixed together in these savory muffins. In the end, you'll have something that pleases everyone, kids to grown-ups. Jarred pizza sauce often contains a large quantity of sugar and oil, so we prefer plain tomato sauce and fresh spices. These muffins can make a great lunch alongside a salad. They're also terrific on picnics.

Nonstick spray or paper muffin cups
1/4 cup olive oil
1 medium onion, finely chopped
1 medium green bell pepper, cored, seeded, and finely chopped
8 ounces cremini mushrooms, cleaned and thinly sliced
1 2/3 cups all-purpose flour
2 tablespoons sugar
1 tablespoon baking powder
2 large eggs, lightly beaten, at room temperature
One 8-ounce can tomato sauce
2/3 cup grated Parmigiano-Reggiano (a little less than 4 ounces)
2 teaspoons chopped fresh rosemary
2 teaspoons chopped fresh oregano
1/2 teaspoon garlic powder
1/2 teaspoon salt (optional)

1. Position the rack in the center of the oven and preheat the oven to 400°F. To prepare the muffin tins, spray the indentations and the rims around them with nonstick spray, or line the indentations with paper muffin cups. If using silicon muffin tins, spray as directed, then place them on a baking sheet.

2. Heat a large skillet over medium heat, then swirl in the oil. Add the onion, green pepper, and mushrooms; cook, stirring frequently, for about 4 minutes, or until the mushrooms have given off their liquid and it has evaporated. Transfer the contents of the skillet to a large bowl; cool for 5 minutes.

3. Meanwhile, whisk the flour, sugar, and baking powder in a small bowl until well combined. Set aside.

4. Stir the eggs, tomato sauce, cheese, rosemary, oregano, garlic powder, and salt into the vegetables. Then stir in the flour mixture until incorporated.

5. Fill the prepared tins three-quarters full. Use additional greased tins or individual, ovensafe, greased ramekins for any leftover batter, or reserve the batter for a second baking. For best results, make sure any vegetables are submerged in the batter, not sticking out of the top of the muffins. Bake for 23 minutes, or until the muffins have well rounded, lightly browned tops and a toothpick inserted in the center of one muffin comes out clean, provided the vegetables don't gum it up.

6. Set the pan on a wire rack to cool for 10 minutes. Gently tip each muffin to one side to make sure it isn't stuck. If one is, gently rock it back and forth to release it from the tin. Remove the muffins and cool for 5 minutes more on the rack before serving. If storing or freezing the muffins, cool them completely before sealing in an airtight container or in freezer-safe plastic bags. The muffins will stay fresh for up to 2 days at room temperature or up to 2 months in the freezer.

> **Pepperoni Pizza Muffins:** *Omit the mushrooms. Add 1/4 cup coarsely chopped pepperoni with the tomato sauce.*
>
> **Sausage Pizza Muffins:** *Omit the mushrooms. Reduce the olive oil to 2 tablespoons. Add 6 ounces crumbled Italian pork sausage meat to the skillet with the onions; cook until the sausage is browned, stirring frequently. Drain all but 2 tablespoons fat from the skillet before adding its contents to the large bowl.*

Poppy Seed Muffins

Makes 12 muffins

Unlike in Lemon Poppy Seed Muffins (page 108), poppy seeds here stand on their own in these light, moist muffins, tangy with sour cream. Just as with poppy seed bagels, these are perfect smeared with softened cream cheese.

Nonstick spray or paper muffin cups

$^1/_2$ **cup poppy seeds**

4 tablespoons ($^1/_2$ stick) unsalted butter, melted and cooled

2$^1/_4$ cups all-purpose flour

2 teaspoons baking soda

1 teaspoon baking powder

$^1/_2$ **teaspoon salt**

2 large eggs, at room temperature

$^3/_4$ **cup sugar**

$^1/_2$ **cup milk (whole, low-fat, or nonfat)**

1 cup sour cream (regular, low-fat, or nonfat)

2 tablespoons Amaretto liqueur, or other almond-flavored liqueur, or
  2 tablespoons Grade A Dark Amber maple syrup

1 teaspoon vanilla extract

1. Position the rack in the center of the oven and preheat the oven to 400°F. To prepare the muffin tins, spray the indentations and the rims around them with nonstick spray, or line the indentations with paper muffin cups. If using silicon muffin tins, spray as directed, then place them on a baking sheet.

2. Stir the poppy seeds and butter in a small bowl until blended, then set aside for 5 minutes to allow the poppy seeds to soften slightly.

3. Meanwhile, whisk the flour, baking soda, baking powder, and salt in a medium bowl until uniform. Set aside.

4. In a large bowl, whisk the eggs and sugar until smooth and pale yellow, about 2 minutes. Whisk in the milk until smooth, then whisk in the sour cream, Amaretto or maple syrup, and vanilla. Use a wooden spoon to stir in the poppy seeds and any but-

ter left in the bowl, and then add the flour mixture, stirring just until the poppy seeds and flour are evenly distributed in the batter. Do not overmix.

5. Fill the prepared tins three-quarters full. Use additional greased tins or individual, ovensafe, greased ramekins for any leftover batter, or reserve the batter for a second baking. Bake for 22 minutes, or until the muffins are golden brown with rounded, cracked tops. A toothpick inserted into the center of one muffin should come out with a few moist crumbs attached.

6. Set the pan on a wire rack to cool for 10 minutes. Gently rock each muffin back and forth to release and remove it from the tin. Cool them for 5 minutes more on the rack before serving. If storing or freezing the muffins, cool them completely before sealing in an airtight container or in freezer-safe plastic bags. The muffins will stay fresh for up to 24 hours at room temperature or up to 1 month in the freezer.

Poppy Seed Oat Crunch Muffins: *Top the muffins with Oat Crunch Topping (page 230) before serving.*

Poppy Seed Orange Muffins: *Add 2 tablespoons grated orange zest with the sour cream.*

Poppy Seed Pecan Muffins: *Mix 1/2 cup chopped pecans with the flour.*

Potato Muffins

Makes 12 muffins

Reminiscent of the potato rolls sold in Portuguese bakeries, these mashed potato muffins are neither light-as-air nor dense-as-dumplings. Instead, they're satisfying enough to serve alongside a bowl of tomato soup but tender enough to complement a sliced tomato salad.

1 pound russet baking potatoes, peeled and cut into 1-inch pieces
Nonstick spray or paper muffin cups
2 cups all-purpose flour
1 tablespoon baking powder
1 teaspoon salt
1 cup whole milk
1/2 cup sour cream (regular, low-fat, or nonfat)
1 tablespoon Dijon mustard
1 large egg, lightly beaten, at room temperature

1. Place the potatoes in a medium saucepan; cover them with cold water by 2 inches. Bring the water to a boil over high heat. Reduce the heat to medium-low and simmer for 10 minutes, uncovered, or until the potatoes are tender when pierced with a fork. Drain in a colander in the sink and cool for 10 minutes.

2. Meanwhile, position the rack in the center of the oven and preheat the oven to 400°F. To prepare the muffin tins, spray the indentations and the rims around them with nonstick spray, or line the indentations with paper muffin cups. If using silicon muffin tins, spray as directed, then place them on a baking sheet.

3. Mix the flour, baking powder, and salt in a medium bowl; set aside.

4. Transfer the potatoes to a large bowl; use an electric mixer at medium speed to beat in 1/2 cup of the milk, the sour cream, and the mustard. Continue beating until creamy, about 1 minute, scraping down the sides of the bowl as necessary.

5. Using a rubber spatula, stir in the remaining 1/2 cup milk and the egg until smooth. Stir in 3/4 of the flour mixture, just until incorporated. Add the remaining flour mixture 1 tablespoon at a time until the batter is quite thick but can still be dropped with a wooden spoon.

6. Fill the prepared tins almost to the top. Bake for 30 minutes, or until the muffins have golden, rounded tops. A toothpick inserted in the center of one muffin should come out clean.

7. Set the pan on a wire rack to cool for 10 minutes. Gently rock each muffin back and forth to release and remove it from the tin. Cool them for 5 minutes more on the rack before serving. If storing or freezing the muffins, cool them completely before sealing in an airtight container or in freezer-safe plastic bags. The muffins will stay fresh for up to 24 hours at room temperature or up to 1 month in the freezer.

Buttery Potato Muffins: *Brush the tops of the muffins with melted unsalted butter after baking 20 minutes, then continue baking the remaining 10 minutes.*

Potato Cheddar Muffins: *Add 1/2 cup shredded Cheddar cheese (about 2 ounces) with the milk. Top each muffin with 2 teaspoons shredded Cheddar before baking.*

Potato Chive Muffins: *Add 1/4 cup finely chopped fresh chives with the milk.*

Potato Dill Muffins: *Add 2 tablespoons chopped fresh dill with the milk.*

Prune Muffins

Makes 12 muffins

Rather than soaking prunes for at least 30 minutes to soften them, bakers often use lekvar, made from puréed prunes, as a quick and easy way to create a prune-based batter. Lekvar adds so much moisture to a batter that it's also used as a fat substitute in baking. Look for lekvar (sometimes called prune butter) in the baking aisle of most supermarkets.

Nonstick spray or paper muffin cups
1³/4 cups all-purpose flour
1/2 cup whole wheat flour
2 teaspoons baking soda
1/2 teaspoon baking powder
1/2 teaspoon salt
1 cup lekvar
1 cup packed light brown sugar
1 large egg, at room temperature
1 cup buttermilk (regular or low-fat)
1 teaspoon vanilla extract

1. Position the rack in the center of the oven and preheat the oven to 400°F. To prepare the muffin tins, spray the indentations and the rims around them with nonstick spray, or line the indentations with paper muffin cups. If using silicon muffin tins, spray as directed, then place them on a baking sheet.

2. Whisk the all-purpose flour, whole wheat flour, baking soda, baking powder, and salt in a medium bowl until uniform. Set aside.

3. In a large bowl, whisk the lekvar and brown sugar until smooth. Whisk in the egg until well blended, then whisk in the buttermilk and vanilla extract. Finally, use a wooden spoon to stir in the prepared flour mixture just until moistened.

4. Fill the prepared tins three-quarters full. Use additional greased tins or small, oven-safe, greased ramekins for any leftover batter, or reserve the batter for a second baking. Bake for 20 minutes, or until the muffins have rounded, cracked tops and a

toothpick inserted in the center of one muffin comes out with a crumb or two attached.

5. Set the pan on a wire rack to cool for 10 minutes. Gently rock each muffin back and forth to release and remove it from the tin. Cool them for 5 minutes more on the rack before serving. If storing or freezing, cool the muffins completely before sealing them in an airtight container or in freezer-safe plastic bags. The muffins will stay fresh for up to 24 hours at room temperature or up to 1 month in the freezer.

> **Prune Maple Muffins:** *Reduce the light brown sugar to 1/2 cup. Add 1/2 cup maple sugar with the remaining brown sugar.*
>
> **Prune Nut Muffins:** *Add 3/4 cup chopped, toasted nuts, such as almonds, hazelnuts, pecans, or walnuts, with the flour.*
>
> **Spiced Prune Rum Muffins:** *Add 1 teaspoon ground cinnamon, 1/2 teaspoon ground ginger, and 1/4 teaspoon grated nutmeg with the flour. Stir in 1 teaspoon rum extract with the vanilla.*

Pumpkin Muffins

Makes 12 muffins

Canned pumpkin is a bit of a misnomer. There's rarely pumpkin in it at all—instead, what's used is usually the large, orange-fleshed, blue hubbard squash. According to FDA guidelines (issued in 1969 and again in 1988), packers are allowed to label a can "pumpkin," even if it's 100 percent blue hubbard squash. Regardless, canned pumpkin adds that characteristic pumpkin taste to recipes, including this one, for moist, dense muffins. Use solid-pack pumpkin, not canned pumpkin pie filling, which contains extra sugar and spices. And see what your friends say when you present them with Blue Hubbard Squash Muffins!

Nonstick spray or paper muffin cups
2^1/$_2$ cups all-purpose flour
^{1}/$_4$ cup granulated sugar
2 teaspoons baking powder
1 teaspoon baking soda
^{1}/$_2$ teaspoon ground cinnamon
^{1}/$_2$ teaspoon salt
2 large eggs, at room temperature
^{3}/$_4$ cup packed dark brown sugar
One 15-ounce can solid-pack pumpkin (about 1^1/$_2$ cups canned pumpkin)
^{3}/$_4$ cup buttermilk (regular or low-fat)
6 tablespoons (^{3}/$_4$ stick) unsalted butter, melted and cooled
1 teaspoon vanilla extract

1. Position the rack in the center of the oven and preheat the oven to 400°F. To prepare the muffin tins, spray the indentations and the rims around them with nonstick spray, or line the indentations with paper muffin cups. If using silicon muffin tins, spray as directed, then place them on a baking sheet.

2. Whisk the flour, granulated sugar, baking powder, baking soda, cinnamon, and salt in a medium bowl until well combined. Set aside.

3. In a large bowl, whisk the eggs until lightly beaten, then whisk in the brown sugar. Continue whisking until the mixture is thick and pale brown, about 2 minutes.

Whisk in the pumpkin, buttermilk, melted butter, and vanilla extract. Once the mixture is smooth, stir in the prepared flour mixture until incorporated. Do not overmix.

4. Fill the prepared tins three-quarters full. Use additional greased tins or small, oven-safe, greased ramekins for any leftover batter, or reserve the batter for a second baking. Bake for 22 minutes, or until the muffins are dark brown with rounded, cracked tops. A toothpick inserted into the center of one muffin should come out with a few moist crumbs attached.

5. Set the pan on a wire rack to cool for 10 minutes. Gently rock each muffin back and forth to release and remove it from the tin. Cool them for 5 minutes more on the rack before serving. If storing or freezing, cool the muffins completely before sealing them in an airtight container or in freezer-safe plastic bags. The muffins will stay fresh for up to 24 hours at room temperature or up to 1 month in the freezer.

> **Cranberry Pumpkin Muffins:** *Add 1/2 cup dried cranberries with the pumpkin.*
>
> **Marshmallow Nut Pumpkin Muffins:** *Add 1/2 cup mini marshmallows and 1/2 cup chopped, toasted pecans with the flour.*
>
> **Orange Pecan Pumpkin Muffins:** *Add 2 teaspoons grated orange zest and 1/2 cup chopped, toasted pecans with the pumpkin.*
>
> **Pumpkin Seed Pumpkin Muffins:** *Add 1/2 cup toasted shelled pumpkin seeds (pepitás) with the flour.*
>
> **Spiced Pumpkin Muffins:** *Increase the cinnamon to 1 teaspoon. Add 1/4 teaspoon grated nutmeg, 1/4 teaspoon ground mace, and 1/2 teaspoon ground ginger with the cinnamon.*

Quiche Lorraine Muffins

Makes 12 muffins

Call it the best way to combine the '80s and the '90s—a quiche craze fused with a muffin craze. Quiche Lorraine has always been the best of all quiches: packed with bacon and Gruyère, a hard cheese that melts to perfection. The best part about these muffins? They're hearty enough to be a meal with a salad and glass of wine or iced tea.

Nonstick spray or paper muffin cups
$^1/_4$ cup canola or vegetable oil
6 strips thick-cut bacon, or 8 thin strips bacon, roughly chopped
4 medium scallions, thinly sliced
2 cups all-purpose flour
$^1/_2$ cup yellow or white cornmeal
1 tablespoon baking powder
1 tablespoon sugar
$^1/_2$ teaspoon salt
1 large egg, at room temperature
2 large egg yolks, at room temperature
1 cup whole milk
$1^1/_4$ cups shredded Gruyère (5 ounces)

1. Position the rack in the center of the oven and preheat the oven to 400°F. To prepare the muffin tins, spray the indentations and the rims around them with nonstick spray, or line the indentations with paper muffin cups. If using silicon muffin tins, spray as directed, then place them on a baking sheet.

2. Heat a medium skillet over medium heat. Swirl in 1 tablespoon of the oil, then add the bacon and sauté for 1 minute. Add the scallions and cook for 2 minutes, stirring occasionally, until the scallions are wilted and the bacon is lightly browned. Transfer the contents of the skillet to a large bowl and cool for 10 minutes.

3. Meanwhile, whisk the flour, cornmeal, baking powder, sugar, and salt in a medium bowl until well blended. Set aside.

4. Whisk the egg, egg yolks, and the remaining oil into the bowl with the bacon. Stir in the milk and cheese until well incorporated. Finally, stir in the prepared flour mixture until moistened.

5. Fill the prepared tins three-quarters full. Use additional greased tins or small, oven-safe, greased ramekins for any leftover batter, or reserve the batter for a second baking. Bake for 18 minutes, or until the muffins are lightly browned and a toothpick inserted in the center of one muffin comes out with a few moist crumbs attached.

6. Set the pan on a wire rack to cool for 10 minutes. Gently tip each muffin to one side to make sure it isn't stuck. If one is, rock it back and forth to release it from the tin. Remove the muffins and cool them for 5 minutes more on the rack before serving. If storing or freezing, cool them completely before sealing them in an airtight container or in freezer-safe plastic bags. The muffins will stay fresh for up to 2 days at room temperature or up to 3 months in the freezer.

> **Duck Confit Quiche Lorraine Muffins:** *Omit the bacon. Remove the fat from 1 large duck confit leg (about 6 ounces). Place the fat in the skillet over medium heat. When it's melted, shred the meat off the leg and add it to the skillet with the scallions. Sauté for 3 minutes, or until the scallions are wilted, stirring frequently.*
>
> **Mushroom Quiche Lorraine Muffins:** *Omit the bacon. Add 1 1/2 cups thinly sliced mushrooms to the skillet with the scallions. Sauté for 4 minutes, or until the mushrooms give off their liquid and it evaporates.*
>
> **Smoked Turkey Quiche Lorraine Muffins:** *Omit the bacon. Add 1 cup chopped smoked turkey to the skillet with the scallions.*

Red Velvet Muffins

Makes 12 muffins

Although a staple of Southern cooking, red velvet cake was first created at New York's Waldorf Astoria hotel, a symbol of the good life, access to which was only on the other side of red velvet ropes. In honor of the good life, these light-as-air chocolate muffins are stained velvet red with lots of food coloring—an entire bottle, in fact, which may seem excessive, but is necessary to give these muffins their characteristic hue.

Nonstick spray or paper muffin cups
2 cups all-purpose flour
1^1/4 cups sugar
1/4 cup cocoa powder, sifted
2^1/2 teaspoons baking soda
1/2 teaspoon salt
1 large egg, at room temperature
1^1/3 cups buttermilk (regular or low-fat)
8 tablespoons (1 stick) unsalted butter, melted and cooled
2 teaspoons vanilla extract
2 teaspoons white vinegar
One ^{1}/2-ounce bottle red food coloring

1. Position the rack in the center of the oven and preheat the oven to 400°F. To prepare the muffin tins, spray the indentations and the rims around them with nonstick spray, or line the indentations with paper muffin cups. If using silicon muffin tins, spray as directed, then place the tins on a baking sheet.

2. Whisk the flour, sugar, cocoa powder, baking soda, and salt in a medium bowl until uniform. Set aside.

3. In a large bowl, lightly whisk the egg, then whisk in the buttermilk and melted butter until smooth. Whisk in the vanilla, vinegar, and red food coloring until the mixture is uniformly colored. Use a wooden spoon to stir in the flour mixture, just until moistened.

4. Fill the prepared tins three-quarters full. Use additional greased tins or small, oven-safe, greased ramekins for any leftover batter, or reserve the batter for a second bak-

ing. Bake for 27 minutes, or until the tops are browned and cracked and a toothpick inserted in the center of one muffin comes out with a few moist crumbs attached.

5. Set the pan on a wire rack to cool for 10 minutes. Gently rock each muffin back and forth to release and remove it from the tin. Cool the muffins for 5 minutes more on the rack before serving. If storing or freezing them, cool them completely before sealing in an airtight container or in freezer-safe plastic bags. The muffins will stay fresh for up to 24 hours at room temperature, or up to 1 month in the freezer.

Red Velvet Cherry Muffins: *Add 1/2 cup dried cherries with the flour.*

Red Velvet Chocolate Chip Muffins: *Add 1/2 cup semisweet chocolate chips with the flour.*

Red Velvet Mint Chip Muffins: *Omit the vinegar. Add 1/2 cup milk chocolate chips with the flour. Stir in 1 teaspoon mint extract with the vanilla.*

Red Velvet Nut Muffins: *Stir in 1/2 cup toasted nuts, such as sliced almond, chopped pecans, or chopped walnuts, with the flour.*

Red Velvet Peanut Butter Chip Muffins: *Omit the vinegar. Add 1/2 cup peanut butter chips flavored with the flour.*

Red Velvet Vanilla Glazed Muffins: *Coat the cooled muffins with Vanilla Dip (page 231).*

Refrigerator Honey Bran Muffins

Makes about 3 dozen muffins

Refrigerator muffins are a holiday tradition in many homes—and should be in all. You just whip up a batter and keep it, tightly covered, in the refrigerator for up to 4 weeks; scoop out as much as you need, for as many muffins as you want, and bake it at will. Bran and a high acidity help keep the batter from fermenting during storage, but use the freshest ingredients to ensure the best shelf life. These muffins are sweet and moist, thanks to loads of honey and buttermilk.

3 cups All-Bran cereal

1 cup wheat bran (do not use bran cereal)

2 cups boiling water

3 large eggs, lightly beaten

3 cups buttermilk (regular or low-fat)

$^3/4$ cup sugar

$^3/4$ cup packed light brown sugar

$^3/4$ cup honey

$^3/4$ cup canola or vegetable oil

4 cups all-purpose flour

$1^1/2$ tablespoons baking soda

$1^1/2$ teaspoons ground cinnamon

1 teaspoon salt

Nonstick spray or paper muffin cups

1. Place the cereal and bran in a very large bowl; pour in the boiling water. Mix until moist and uniform, then cool for 15 minutes. Make sure the mixture is smooth—mash out any clumps of bran before proceeding.

2. Whisk the eggs, buttermilk, sugar, brown sugar, honey, and oil in a medium bowl until smooth. Mix into the bran mixture, preferably using your hands or a large wooden spoon. Make sure to stir out any lumps. Then mix in the flour, baking soda, cinnamon, and salt until well combined.

3. Store the batter, tightly sealed, in the refrigerator for up to 1 month.

4. To bake, position the rack in the center of the oven and preheat the oven to 375°F. Spray the indentations of a muffin tin and the rims around them with nonstick spray, or line the indentations with paper muffin cups. If using silicon muffin tins, spray as directed, then place them on a baking sheet.

5. Spoon the batter into the cups until they are three-quarters full. Reseal the remaining batter and store it in the refrigerator.

6. Bake the muffins for 25 minutes, or until the tops are browned and nicely rounded. A toothpick inserted into the center of one muffin should come out with a few moist crumbs attached.

7. Cool the muffins in their tin on a wire rack for 10 minutes, then remove the muffins and continue cooling on the rack for another 5 minutes.

Mix in any of the following, or any combination of the following, with the flour:

1 tablespoon vanilla extract
2 teaspoons ground ginger
1 teaspoon grated nutmeg
1 teaspoon ground mace

Refrigerator Oat Bran Muffins

Makes about 4 dozen muffins

These are classic bran muffins—fairly heavy, but with a brilliant wake-me-up taste, thanks to the oat bran. They bake up dark and very moist and slightly less sweet than the Refrigerator Honey Bran Muffins (page 180). Still warm from the oven, all they need is a pat of butter.

> **3 cups All-Bran cereal**
> **1³/4 cups wheat bran (do not use bran cereal)**
> **1³/4 cups oat bran**
> **1 cup rolled oats (do not use quick-cooking oats)**
> **5 cups boiling water**
> **4 large eggs, lightly beaten**
> **4 cups buttermilk (regular or low-fat)**
> **1 cup canola or vegetable oil**
> **¹/2 cup unsulphured molasses**
> **4 cups all-purpose flour**
> **2¹/2 cups sugar**
> **3 tablespoons baking soda**
> **2 teaspoons salt**
> **Nonstick spray or paper muffin cups**

1. Place the cereal, wheat bran, oat bran, and rolled oats in a very large bowl; pour the boiling water over them. Mix until moist and uniform, then cool for about 15 minutes. Mash out any clumps of bran with the back of a wooden spoon before proceeding.

2. Whisk the eggs, buttermilk, oil, and molasses in a medium bowl until smooth. Pour this mixture into the bran mixture; mix together, preferably using your hands or a large wooden spoon. Stir out any lumps. Then mix in the flour, sugar, baking soda, and salt, until well combined.

3. Store the batter, tightly sealed, in the refrigerator for up to 1 month.

4. To bake, position the rack in the center of the oven and preheat the oven to 375°F. Spray the indentations of a muffin tin and the rims around them with nonstick

spray, or line the indentations with paper muffin cups. If using silicon muffin tins, spray as directed, then place them on a baking sheet.

5. Spoon the batter into the cups until three-quarters full. Reseal any remaining batter and store it in the refrigerator.

6. Bake the muffins for 25 minutes, or until the nicely rounded tops are deeply browned. A toothpick inserted into the center of one muffin should come out clean.

7. Cool the muffins in their tin on a wire rack for 10 minutes, then remove the muffins and continue cooling on the rack for another 5 minutes before serving.

Before baking, scoop out as much batter as you need. Mix in any of the following, individually or in combination, to equal the total volume based on the chart below.

Chopped dried apricots • Dried blueberries • Mini semisweet chocolate chips • Peanut butter chips • Pine nuts • Raisins • Shelled, unsalted pistachios • Sliced almonds • Sliced bananas • Sunflower seeds • Toasted chopped hazelnuts • Toasted pecan pieces • Toasted sliced almonds • Toasted walnut pieces

If you're making	Add
1 muffin	1 tablespoon of the above, or any combination of the above
3 muffins	3 tablespoons
4 muffins	1/4 cup
5 muffins	1/3 cup
6 muffins	1/4 cup plus 2 tablespoons
8 muffins	1/2 cup
10 muffins	2/3 cup
12 muffins	3/4 cup

Rice Flour Muffins

Makes 12 muffins

These muffins are perfect for gluten-free diets. They're great with butter and jam, or can be gussied up with the variations below. The white rice flour makes them moist and light, especially since it's combined with tapioca flour and xanthan gum (for more on xanthan gum, see page 95). Look for all these ingredients in health food stores or the baking aisle of some gourmet markets.

> **Nonstick spray or paper muffin cups**
> **1³/4 cups white rice flour**
> **1/4 cup tapioca flour**
> **2 teaspoons baking soda**
> **1 teaspoon ground cinnamon**
> **1/2 teaspoon baking powder, or gluten-free baking powder**
> **1/2 teaspoon xanthan gum**
> **1/2 teaspoon salt**
> **2 large eggs, separated, at room temperature**
> **1/2 cup packed dark brown sugar**
> **1/2 cup yogurt (regular, low-fat, or nonfat)**
> **1/2 cup milk (whole, low-fat, or nonfat)**
> **6 tablespoons (³/4 stick) unsalted butter, melted and cooled**
> **2 teaspoons vanilla extract, or gluten-free vanilla extract**

1. Position the rack in the center of the oven and preheat the oven to 400°F. To prepare the muffin tins, spray the indentations and the rims around them with nonstick spray, or line the indentations with paper muffin cups. If using silicon muffin tins, spray as directed, then place the tins on a baking sheet.

2. Whisk the rice flour, tapioca flour, baking soda, cinnamon, baking powder, xanthan gum, and salt in a small bowl until well combined. Set aside.

3. Place the egg whites in a medium bowl and beat them with an electric mixer at high speed until stiff but not dry peaks form. Set aside as well.

4. In a large bowl, whisk the egg yolks and brown sugar until thick and pale brown, about 2 minutes. Whisk in the yogurt, milk, melted butter, and vanilla until smooth.

5. Use a rubber spatula to stir in the rice flour mixture until incorporated. Then gently fold in the beaten egg whites. There will be white streaks in the batter.

6. Fill the prepared tins three-quarters full. Use additional greased tins or small, oven-safe, greased ramekins for any leftover batter, or reserve the batter for a second baking. Bake for 16 minutes, or until the tops are set but spongy, and a toothpick inserted in the center of one muffin comes out clean.

7. Set the pan on a wire rack to cool for 10 minutes. Gently rock each muffin back and forth to release and remove it from the tin. Cool the muffins for 5 minutes more on the rack before serving. If storing or freezing them, cool them completely before sealing in an airtight container or in freezer-safe plastic bags. The muffins will stay fresh for up to 24 hours at room temperature or up to 1 month in the freezer.

> **Rice Flour Almond Muffins:** *Add 1/2 teaspoon almond extract with the vanilla. Top each muffin with 1 teaspoon sliced almonds before baking.*
>
> **Rice Flour Apricot Pistachio Muffins:** *Add 1/2 cup chopped dried apricots and 1/4 cup chopped, shelled, unsalted pistachios with the rice flour.*
>
> **Rice Flour Chocolate Chip Muffins:** *Add 2/3 cup semisweet chocolate chips with the rice flour.*
>
> **Rice Flour Cranberry Muffins:** *Add 2/3 cup dried cranberries with the rice flour.*
>
> **Rice Flour Pecan Muffins:** *Add 2/3 cup chopped pecan pieces with the rice flour.*
>
> **Rice Flour Raisin Muffins:** *Add 2/3 cup regular or golden raisins with the rice flour.*

Rice Pudding Muffins

Makes 12 muffins

These muffins are an easy way to use up leftover rice, either from dinner or Chinese take-out the night before. Just make sure the rice hasn't been salted or flavored before you use it. The resulting muffins are decadent and creamy, just like rice pudding.

Nonstick spray or paper muffin cups
$1^1/4$ cups cooked white rice
$1/2$ cup heavy cream
4 tablespoons ($1/2$ stick) unsalted butter, melted and cooled
$1^1/2$ cups all-purpose flour
$2/3$ cup sugar
1 tablespoon baking powder
$1/2$ teaspoon grated nutmeg
$1/2$ teaspoon salt
1 large egg, at room temperature
1 cup milk (whole, low-fat, or nonfat)
$3/4$ cup chopped dried cherries
1 teaspoon vanilla extract

1. Position the rack in the center of the oven and preheat the oven to 400°F. To prepare the muffin tins, spray the indentations and the rims around them with nonstick spray, or line the indentations with paper muffin cups. If using silicon muffin tins, spray as directed, then place the tins on a baking sheet.

2. Combine the rice, cream, and melted butter in a large bowl, stir well, then set aside for 10 minutes.

3. Meanwhile, whisk the flour, sugar, baking powder, nutmeg, and salt in a medium bowl until well combined. Set aside.

4. Whisk the egg and milk in a small bowl until smooth; stir this egg mixture into the rice mixture. Stir in the dried cherries and vanilla extract until well blended. Finally, stir in the prepared flour mixture until the rice and cherries are evenly distributed in the batter. Do not overmix.

5. Fill the prepared tins three-quarters full. Use additional greased tins or small, oven-safe, greased ramekins for any leftover batter, or reserve the batter for a second baking. Bake for 22 minutes, or until the muffins are well browned and a toothpick inserted in the center of one muffin comes out clean.

6. Set the pan on a wire rack to cool for 10 minutes. Gently rock each muffin back and forth to release and remove it from the tin. Cool the muffins for 5 minutes more on the rack before serving. If storing or freezing them, cool them completely before sealing in an airtight container or in freezer-safe plastic bags. The muffins will stay fresh for up to 2 days at room temperature or up to 2 months in the freezer.

Almond Rice Pudding Muffins: *Add 1/2 cup toasted slivered almonds with the dried cherries. Add 1/2 teaspoon almond extract with the vanilla.*

Banana Rice Pudding Muffins: *Substitute chopped dried banana for the dried cherries.*

Chocolate Rice Pudding Muffins: *Substitute semisweet chocolate chips for the dried cherries. Top the cooled muffins with Chocolate Icing (page 223).*

Ginger Rice Pudding Muffins: *Reduce the dried cherries to 1/2 cup. Add 1/3 cup chopped crystallized ginger with the remaining cherries.*

Lemon Glazed Rice Pudding Muffins: *Top the muffins with Lemon Drizzle (page 227).*

Raisin Rice Pudding Muffins: *Substitute golden raisins for the dried cherries.*

Vanilla Glazed Rice Pudding Muffins: *Coat the cooled muffins with Vanilla Dip (page 231).*

Roasted Garlic Muffins

Makes 12 muffins

Don't think we've lost our minds. When roasted, garlic mellows and sweetens considerably. Here, it's folded into savory muffins which will lend themselves to most dinners, from roasts to casseroles. If you'd like, serve them with a bowl of extra virgin olive oil for dipping.

> **1 medium garlic head (about 3 ounces)**
> **$1/4$ cup plus 1 tablespoon olive oil**
> **Nonstick spray or paper muffin cups**
> **2 large eggs, at room temperature**
> **$3/4$ cup milk (whole, low-fat, or nonfat)**
> **$3/4$ cup small-curd cottage cheese, or cream-style cottage cheese (regular or low-fat, but not nonfat)**
> **$1^1/2$ cups all-purpose flour**
> **$1/2$ cup whole wheat flour**
> **$1/4$ cup grated Parmigiano-Reggiano (about 1 ounce)**
> **2 tablespoons sugar**
> **1 tablespoon baking powder**
> **$1/2$ teaspoon salt**

1. Position the rack in the center of the oven and preheat the oven to 400°F.

2. Cut the top quarter off the garlic head so that the cloves are exposed. Discard the top quarter. Place the garlic on a small sheet of aluminum foil, drizzle with 1 tablespoon of the olive oil, then fold and seal the sides of the foil to create a pouch around the garlic. Place directly on the oven rack and bake for about 35 minutes, or until the garlic smells sweet and the cloves are soft. Remove from the oven and cool for 15 minutes without unwrapping. Maintain the oven's temperature.

3. To prepare the muffin tins, spray the indentations and the rims around them with nonstick spray, or line the indentations with paper muffin cups. If using silicon muffin tins, spray as directed, then place the tins on a baking sheet.

4. Squeeze the cooled pulp from the garlic cloves into a large bowl, discarding the papery husks. Mash the garlic with a fork, then whisk in the eggs, milk, cottage

cheese, and remaining 1/4 cup of the olive oil. Set aside for 10 minutes to infuse the garlic flavor into the mixture.

5. Whisk the all-purpose flour, whole wheat flour, Parmigiano-Reggiano, sugar, baking powder, and salt in a small bowl until uniform. Stir this dry mixture into the garlic mixture with a wooden spoon until moistened.

6. Fill the prepared tins three-quarters full. Use additional greased tins or small, oven-safe, greased ramekins for any leftover batter, or reserve the batter for a second baking. Bake for 20 minutes, or until the muffins have lightly browned, rounded tops and a toothpick inserted in the center of one muffin comes out with a crumb or two attached.

7. Set the pan on a wire rack to cool for 10 minutes. Gently rock each muffin back and forth to release and remove it from the tin. Cool the muffins for 5 minutes more on the rack before serving. If storing or freezing them, cool them completely before sealing in an airtight container or in freezer-safe plastic bags. The muffins will stay fresh for up to 24 hours at room temperature or up to 1 month in the freezer.

> **Roasted Garlic Basil Muffins:** *Add 2 tablespoons chopped fresh basil with the eggs.*
>
> **Roasted Garlic Pine Nut Muffins:** *Add 1/2 cup toasted pine nuts with the flour.*
>
> **Roasted Garlic Prosciutto Muffins:** *Add 1/2 cup finely chopped prosciutto with the eggs.*
>
> **Roasted Garlic Provolone Muffins:** *Omit the Parmigiano-Reggiano. Add 1/2 cup finely diced provolone (about 2 ounces) with the eggs.*
>
> **Roasted Garlic Sun-Dried Tomato Muffins:** *Add 2/3 cup finely chopped, drained, marinated sun-dried tomatoes with the eggs.*

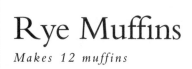

Rye Muffins

Makes 12 muffins

Rye flour is too heavy and has too few glutens to work successfully in quick breads, so the trick is to use rye flakes, which give muffins that distinctive rye taste without weighing them down. Look for rye flakes in health food stores and in many gourmet markets. These savory muffins are a little chewy and very aromatic, just the right accompaniment to soups or main-course salads.

Nonstick spray or paper muffin cups
1^{1}/3 cups rye flakes
1^{1}/4 cups milk (whole, low-fat, or nonfat)
1^{1}/4 cups all-purpose flour
2 teaspoons baking powder
1 teaspoon caraway seeds
1 teaspoon salt
2 large eggs, at room temperature
^{1}/3 cup canola or vegetable oil
1 tablespoon packed light brown sugar
1 teaspoon Dijon mustard

1. Position the rack in the center of the oven and preheat the oven to 400°F. To prepare the muffin tins, spray the indentations and the rims around them with nonstick spray, or line the indentations with paper muffin cups. If using silicon muffin tins, spray as directed, then place the tins on a baking sheet.

2. Place the rye flakes in a large bowl and pour 1/2 cup of the milk over them. Set aside to soften for 5 minutes.

3. Meanwhile, whisk the flour, baking powder, caraway seeds, and salt in a small bowl until uniform. Set aside.

4. Whisk the eggs and the remaining 3/4 cup milk into the bowl with the rye flakes. Whisk in the oil, brown sugar, and mustard until smooth. Let this mixture rest another 5 minutes to infuse the flavors.

5. Stir in the flour mixture until moistened.

6. Fill the prepared tins three-quarters full. Use additional greased tins or small, oven-safe, greased ramekins for any leftover batter, or reserve the batter for a second baking. Bake for 22 minutes, or until the muffins have rounded, cracked tops and a toothpick inserted in the center of one muffin comes out clean.

7. Set the pan on a wire rack to cool for 10 minutes. Gently rock each muffin back and forth to release and remove it from the tin. Cool the muffins for 5 minutes more on the rack before serving. If storing or freezing them, cool them completely before sealing in an airtight container or in freezer-safe plastic bags. The muffins will stay fresh for up to 24 hours at room temperature or up to 1 month in the freezer.

> **Butter-Topped Rye Muffins:** *Melt 3 tablespoons unsalted butter. Brush evenly over the tops of the muffins after they have baked for 15 minutes. Continue baking as directed.*

Sesame Muffins

Makes 12 muffins

Sesame lovers, look no further for your fix. These muffins pack in the flavor of sesame in three ways: 1) with white sesame seeds, often available in the spice section of your supermarket or in bulk at many health food stores; 2) with tahini, a sesame paste used in many Middle Eastern dishes; and 3) with toasted sesame oil, that dark, potent condiment essential to much Asian cooking (not to be confused with the pale, light sesame oil, pressed from untoasted seeds). Buy tahini in a jar rather than a can which is not resealable; store it and the toasted sesame oil in the refrigerator for up to 4 months.

1/4 cup white sesame seeds

Nonstick spray or paper muffin cups

2 cups all-purpose flour

1 tablespoon baking powder

1/2 teaspoon salt

2 large eggs, at room temperature

2/3 cup packed light brown sugar

1 cup milk (whole, low-fat, or nonfat)

1/2 cup tahini

1/4 cup canola or vegetable oil

1 teaspoon toasted sesame oil

1 teaspoon vanilla extract

1. Position the rack in the center of the oven and preheat the oven to 400°F.

2. Spread the sesame seeds evenly across a baking sheet; bake for about 5 minutes, stirring often, until the seeds are light brown and fragrant. Cool for 5 minutes.

3. To prepare the muffin tins, spray the indentations and the rims around them with nonstick spray, or line the indentations with paper muffin cups. If using silicon muffin tins, spray as directed, then place the tins on a baking sheet.

4. In a medium bowl, whisk the flour, baking powder, salt, and the toasted sesame seeds until well combined. Set aside.

5. In a large bowl, whisk the eggs until lightly beaten, then whisk in the brown sugar. Continue whisking until the mixture is thick and pale brown, about 2 minutes.

Whisk in the milk, tahini, canola oil, sesame oil, and vanilla until well blended. Use a wooden spoon to stir in the flour mixture until the sesame seeds are distributed evenly throughout the batter. Do not overmix.

6. Fill the prepared tins three-quarters full. Use additional greased tins or small, oven-safe, greased ramekins for any leftover batter, or reserve the batter for a second baking. Bake for 20 minutes, or until the muffins are lightly browned with rounded, cracked tops. A toothpick inserted into the center of one muffin should come out with a few moist crumbs attached.

7. Set the pan on a wire rack to cool for 10 minutes. Gently rock each muffin back and forth to release and remove it from the tin. Cool the muffins for 5 minutes more on the rack before serving. If storing or freezing them, cool them completely before sealing in an air-tight container or freezer-safe plastic bags. The muffins will stay fresh for up to 24 hours at room temperature or up to 1 month in the freezer.

> **Sesame Candy Muffins:** *Omit the sesame seeds. Add 1/2 cup crushed sesame candy with the flour.*
>
> **Sesame Date Muffins:** *Add 1/2 cup chopped pitted dates with the flour.*
>
> **Sesame Saffron Muffins:** *Add 1/2 teaspoon crumbled saffron threads with the brown sugar.*
>
> **Southwest Sesame Muffins:** *Add 1/4 cup toasted, shelled pumpkin seeds (pepitás) and 1 teaspoon toasted cumin seeds with the milk.*

S'mores Muffins

Makes 12 muffins

Here, the wonderful flavor of the campout favorite jumps right into muffin tins. Graham crackers, marshmallows, and chocolate bake up into a treat worthy of kids of any age. Whip these up for your next bake sale, then stand back and watch the smiles.

Nonstick spray or paper muffin cups
1 cup all-purpose flour
1 cup graham cracker crumbs (see Note)
$1/3$ cup sugar
2 teaspoons baking powder
1 teaspoon baking soda
$1/2$ teaspoon salt
1 large egg, at room temperature
$3/4$ cup yogurt (regular, low-fat, or nonfat)
$3/4$ cup milk (whole, low-fat, or nonfat)
4 tablespoons ($1/2$ stick) unsalted butter, melted and cooled
2 teaspoons vanilla extract
$2/3$ cup semisweet chocolate chips
$3/4$ cup mini marshmallows

1. Position the rack in the center of the oven and preheat the oven to 400°F. To prepare the muffin tins, spray the indentations and the rims around them with nonstick spray, or line the indentations with paper muffin cups. If using silicon muffin tins, spray as directed, then place the tins on a baking sheet.

2. Whisk the flour, graham cracker crumbs, sugar, baking powder, baking soda, and salt in a medium bowl until well blended. Set aside.

3. In a large bowl, whisk the egg until lightly beaten, then whisk in the yogurt until smooth. Whisk in the milk, melted butter, and vanilla extract. Using a wooden spoon, stir in the chocolate chips and mini marshmallows, then stir in the prepared flour mixture until the chips and marshmallows are evenly distributed in the batter. Do not overmix.

4. Fill the prepared tins three-quarters full. Use additional greased tins or small, oven-safe, greased ramekins for any leftover batter, or reserve the batter for a second baking. Bake for 20 minutes, or until the muffins have firm, rounded, lightly browned tops. A toothpick inserted in the center of one muffin should come out with a few moist crumbs attached, provided it doesn't hit a melted chocolate chip and come out too gooey to tell.

5. Set the pan on a wire rack to cool for 10 minutes. Gently tip each muffin to one side to make sure it isn't stuck. If one is, gently rock it back and forth to release it from the tin. Cool the muffins for 5 minutes more on the rack before serving. If storing or freezing them, cool them completely before sealing in an airtight container or in freezer-safe plastic bags. The muffins will stay fresh for up to 2 days at room temperature or up to 2 months in the freezer.

Note: *8 whole graham crackers crushed in a food processor fitted with the chopping blade yield about 1 cup of crumbs.*

> **Chocolate Iced S'mores Muffins:** *Top the cooled muffins with Chocolate Icing (page 223).*
>
> **Peanut S'mores Muffins:** *Reduce the chocolate chips to 1/3 cup. Add 1/3 cup chopped, roasted, unsalted peanuts with the remaining chocolate chips.*
>
> **Rainbow S'mores Muffins:** *Substitute M&M candies for the chocolate chips.*
>
> **White Chocolate Chip S'mores Muffins:** *Substitute white chocolate chips for the semisweet chocolate chips.*

Sour Cream Muffins

Makes 12 muffins

Sour cream makes muffins that are a paradox—creamy yet somehow airy. These muffins are simplicity itself—plain, yes, but they go well with any jam, jelly, marmalade, or honey. They're also fabulous on their own along with a tall glass of iced coffee.

Nonstick spray or paper muffin cups
2 cups all-purpose flour
$^2/_3$ cup sugar
2 teaspoons baking soda
$^1/_2$ teaspoon baking powder
$^1/_2$ teaspoon salt
2 large eggs, at room temperature
1 cup sour cream (regular, low-fat, or nonfat)
$^2/_3$ cup milk (whole, low-fat, or nonfat)
1 teaspoon vanilla extract

1. Position the rack in the center of the oven and preheat the oven to 400°F. To prepare the muffin tins, spray the indentations and the rims around them with nonstick spray, or line the indentations with paper muffin cups. If using silicon muffin tins, spray as directed, then place the tins on a baking sheet.

2. Whisk the flour, sugar, baking soda, baking powder, and salt in a medium bowl until uniform. Set aside.

3. In a large bowl, whisk the eggs and sour cream until smooth, then whisk in the milk and vanilla extract. Stir in the flour mixture with a wooden spoon until incorporated.

4. Fill the prepared tins three-quarters full. Use additional greased tins or small, oven-safe, greased ramekins for any leftover batter, or reserve the batter for a second baking. Bake for 18 minutes, or until the tops are lightly browned but smooth. A toothpick inserted in the center of one muffin should come out with a few moist crumbs attached.

5. Set the pan on a wire rack to cool for 10 minutes. Gently rock each muffin back and forth to release and remove it from the tin. Cool the muffins for 5 minutes more on the rack before serving. If storing or freezing them, cool them completely before sealing in an airtight container or in freezer-safe plastic bags. The muffins will stay fresh for up to 24 hours at room temperature or up to 1 month in the freezer.

Banana Walnut Sour Cream Muffins: *Add 1/2 cup chopped dried banana and 1/2 cup chopped walnuts with the flour.*

Blueberry Sour Cream Muffins: *Add 1 cup dried blueberries with the flour.*

Cherry Sour Cream Muffins: *Add 1 cup dried cherries with the flour.*

Chocolate Chip Sour Cream Muffins: *Add 1 cup semisweet or milk chocolate chips with the flour.*

Chocolate Iced Sour Cream Muffins: *Top the cooled muffins with Chocolate Icing (page 223).*

Cinnamon Crunch Sour Cream Muffins: *Top the muffins with Cinnamon Sugar Topping (page 225) before baking.*

Coconut Sour Cream Muffins: *Add 1 cup sweetened shredded coconut with the flour.*

Cranberry Sour Cream Muffins: *Add 1 cup dried cranberries with the flour.*

Raisin Sour Cream Muffins: *Add 1 cup raisins with the flour.*

Stilton Muffins

Makes 12 muffins

Stilton is one of the best English cheeses, a strong blue cheese made from cow's milk with close to a 50 percent butterfat content. Stilton is traditionally served with walnut bread—so we thought that the combination of rich cheese and toasted nuts would naturally go well in a muffin. Serve these savory gems alongside omelets or steaks.

Nonstick spray or paper muffin cups
1 cup chopped walnut pieces
2 cups all-purpose flour
$^1/_4$ cup sugar
1 tablespoon baking powder
$^1/_4$ teaspoon salt
1 large egg, at room temperature
$1^1/_4$ cups milk (whole or low-fat, but not nonfat)
6 tablespoons ($^3/_4$ stick) unsalted butter, melted and cooled
1 cup crumbled Stilton (about 4 ounces)

1. Position the rack in the center of the oven and preheat the oven to 400°F. To prepare the muffin tins, spray the indentations and the rims around them with nonstick spray, or line the indentations with paper muffin cups. If using silicon muffin tins, spray as directed, then place the tins on a baking sheet.

2. Spread the nuts in a single layer on a baking sheet; bake for about 5 minutes, stirring occasionally, until lightly browned and fragrant. Cool for 5 minutes. Place $^1/_2$ cup of the toasted nuts in a food processor fitted with the chopping blade. Pulse the machine until the nuts are finely ground, but do not grind them into a paste. Place the ground nuts and the reserved walnut pieces, along with the flour, sugar, baking powder, and salt, in a medium bowl. Stir until well combined, then set aside.

3. In a large bowl, whisk the egg until lightly beaten, then whisk in the milk until smooth. Stir in the melted butter and crumbled cheese with a wooden spoon, then stir in the flour mixture until the walnuts and cheese are evenly distributed throughout the batter. Do not overmix.

4. Fill the prepared tins three-quarters full. Use additional greased tins or small, oven-safe, greased ramekins for any leftover batter, or reserve the batter for a second baking. Bake for 23 minutes, or until the muffins are lightly browned with rounded tops. A toothpick inserted in the center of one muffin should come out clean.

5. Set the pan on a wire rack to cool for 10 minutes. Gently tip each muffin to one side to make sure it isn't stuck. If one is, rock it back and forth to release it from the tin. Cool the muffins for 5 minutes more on the rack before serving. Store them in an airtight container once they have cooled completely. The muffins will stay fresh for up to 2 days at room temperature. These muffins do not freeze well.

> **Bacon Stilton Muffins:** *Fry 4 strips of bacon in a skillet with 1 tablespoon canola oil until the bacon is crisp, about 3 minutes, turning the strips once. Drain, then crumble the bacon into the batter with the cheese.*
>
> **Blue Cheese Muffins:** *Substitute any blue cheese for the Stilton, including Danish blue or Gorgonzola.*
>
> **Cherry Stilton Muffins:** *Add 1/3 cup chopped dried cherries with the cheese.*
>
> **Chive Stilton Muffins:** *Add 3 tablespoons chopped fresh chives with the cheese.*
>
> **Corn Stilton Muffins:** *Add 1/2 cup fresh or frozen corn kernels with the cheese.*

Strawberry Jam Muffins

Makes 12 muffins

The batter for these strawberry muffins uses a little oat flour, which, along with the jam, makes them very moist but also a little chewy. They're only as good as the jam you put into them, so buy the best you can comfortably afford. Look for a brand that doesn't use pectin—it does wonders for setting jellies but nothing for muffins. A slightly runny jam, sometimes known as a French-set jam, is preferred.

Nonstick spray or paper muffin cups
1³/4 cups all-purpose flour
¹/2 cup oat flour
¹/3 cup sugar
2 teaspoons baking soda
¹/2 teaspoon baking powder
¹/2 teaspoon salt
2 large eggs, at room temperature
1 cup buttermilk (regular or low-fat)
1 cup strawberry jam (about 10 ounces)
6 tablespoons (³/4 stick) unsalted butter, melted and cooled
1 teaspoon vanilla extract

1. Position the rack in the center of the oven and preheat the oven to 400°F. To prepare the muffin tins, spray the indentations and the rims around them with nonstick spray, or line the indentations with paper muffin cups. If using silicon muffin tins, spray as directed, then place the tins on a baking sheet.

2. Whisk the all-purpose flour, oat flour, sugar, baking soda, baking powder, and salt in a medium bowl until well combined. Set aside.

3. In a large bowl, whisk the eggs until lightly beaten, then whisk in the buttermilk until smooth. Whisk in the jam, melted butter, and vanilla extract. Use a wooden spoon to stir in the prepared flour mixture just until moistened, but make sure that there are no pink streaks in the batter.

4. Fill the prepared tins three-quarters full. Use additional greased tins or small, oven-safe, greased ramekins for any leftover batter, or reserve the batter for a second bak-

ing. Bake for 24 minutes, or until the tops are smooth and browned. A toothpick inserted in the center of one muffin should come out with a few moist crumbs attached.

5. Set the pan on a wire rack to cool for 10 minutes. Gently rock each muffin back and forth to release and remove it from the tin. Cool the muffins for 5 minutes more on the rack before serving. If storing or freezing them, cool them completely before sealing in an airtight container or in freezer-safe plastic bags. The muffins will stay fresh for up to 24 hours at room temperature or up to 1 month in the freezer.

> *You can make an endless variety of jam muffins by simply substituting any other jam for the strawberry jam, including apricot, blackberry, fig, gooseberry, peach, or raspberry.*

Strawberry Muffins

Makes 12 muffins

If you just fold them into a batter, strawberries are simply too wet to make good muffins. And their delicate flavor? Often lost. But if you make a purée using frozen strawberries, the flavor will infuse every crumb. These light, fluffy muffins with a slight pink tint are perfect for a June breakfast—or, thanks to the frozen berries, a December pick-me-up.

Nonstick spray or paper muffin cups

2^1/$_4$ cups all-purpose flour

2 teaspoons baking soda

1 teaspoon baking powder

^{1}/$_2$ teaspoon salt

One 12-ounce package frozen strawberries, thawed

^{2}/$_3$ cup sugar

1 large egg, at room temperature

^{1}/$_2$ cup yogurt (regular, low-fat, or nonfat)

1 teaspoon grated lemon zest

1 teaspoon vanilla extract

1. Position the rack in the center of the oven and preheat the oven to 400°F. To prepare the muffin tins, spray the indentations and the rims around them with nonstick spray, or line the indentations with paper muffin cups. If using silicon muffin tins, spray as directed, then place the tins on a baking sheet.

2. Whisk the flour, baking soda, baking powder, and salt in a large bowl until well combined. Set aside.

3. Place the strawberries, with their juice, and the sugar in a food processor fitted with the chopping blade or in a wide-canister blender. Process for 30 seconds, until the mixture is smooth. Scrape down the sides of the bowl, then add the egg, yogurt, lemon zest, and vanilla. Pulse the machine about 5 times, or until the mixture is blended and uniform.

4. Pour the strawberry mixture over the flour mixture; stir with a wooden spoon until the dry ingredients are incorporated. Do not overmix.

5. Fill the prepared tins three-quarters full. Use additional greased tins or small, oven-safe, greased ramekins for any leftover batter, or reserve the batter for a second baking. Bake for 22 minutes, or until the tops are browned and slightly rounded and a toothpick inserted in the center of one muffin comes out with a crumb or two attached.

6. Set the pan on a wire rack to cool for 10 minutes. Gently rock each muffin back and forth to release and remove it from the tin. Cool the muffins for 5 minutes more on the rack before serving. If storing or freezing them, cool them completely before sealing in an airtight container or in freezer-safe plastic bags. The muffins will stay fresh for up to 24 hours at room temperature or up to 1 month in the freezer.

> **Banana Strawberry Muffins:** *Add 2/3 cup chopped dried banana with the flour.*
>
> **Chocolate Iced Strawberry Muffins:** *Top the cooled muffins with Chocolate Icing (page 223).*
>
> **Coconut Strawberry Muffins:** *Add 1/2 cup sweetened shredded coconut with the flour.*
>
> **Strawberry Cinnamon Crunch Muffins:** *Top the muffins with Cinnamon Sugar Topping (page 225) before baking.*
>
> **Strawberry Crumb Muffins:** *Top the muffins with Crumb Topping (page 226) before baking.*
>
> **Strawberry Malt Muffins:** *Reduce the flour to 2 cups. Add 1/2 cup malted milk powder with the remaining flour.*
>
> **Strawberry Nut Crunch Muffins:** *Top the muffins with Nut Crunch Topping (page 229) before baking.*
>
> **White Chocolate Chip Strawberry Muffins:** *Add 2/3 cup white chocolate chips with the flour.*

Sugar-Free Spelt Muffins

Makes 12 muffins

Spelt is a high-protein grain long favored in the Roman Empire and medieval Europe, but now somewhat out of favor, thanks to the more expeditious production of modern wheat hybrids. Although these muffins are not gluten-free, some people with wheat allergies can tolerate spelt flour. However, we have taken any dairy or sugar out of these muffins, making them just right for a variety of diets. Look for spelt flour in gourmet markets or health food stores.

Nonstick spray for the muffin tins
$1^1/2$ cups spelt flour
$3/4$ cup oat bran
$1^1/2$ teaspoons baking powder
$1/2$ teaspoon baking soda
$1/2$ teaspoon ground cinnamon
$1/2$ teaspoon ground allspice
$1/2$ teaspoon salt
$2/3$ cup dried currants
$1^1/2$ cups unsweetened applesauce
$1/2$ cup unsweetened apple juice
$1/4$ cup plus 1 tablespoon canola or vegetable oil
1 large egg, at room temperature
1 teaspoon vanilla extract

1. Position the rack in the center of the oven and preheat the oven to 400°F. To prepare the muffin tins, spray the indentations and the rims around them with nonstick spray, or line the indentations with paper muffin cups. If using silicon muffin tins, spray as directed, then place the tins on a baking sheet.

2. Whisk the spelt flour, oat bran, baking powder, baking soda, cinnamon, allspice, and salt in a medium bowl until uniform. Add the currants, toss well, and set aside.

3. In a large bowl, whisk the applesauce, apple juice, and oil until smooth; whisk in the egg and vanilla until pale, smooth, and uniform, about 2 minutes. Stir in the spelt mixture with a wooden spoon until incorporated. Let the batter rest for 5 minutes.

4. Fill the prepared tins three-quarters full. Use additional greased tins or small, oven-safe, greased ramekins for any leftover batter, or reserve the batter for a second baking. Bake for 25 minutes, or until the muffins are lightly browned with rounded tops. A toothpick inserted into the center of one muffin should come out clean.

5. Set the pan on a wire rack to cool for 10 minutes. Gently rock each muffin back and forth to release and remove it from the tin. Cool the muffins for 5 minutes more on the rack before serving. If storing or freezing them, cool them completely before sealing in an airtight container or in freezer-safe plastic bags. The muffins will stay fresh for up to 24 hours at room temperature or up to 1 month in the freezer.

> **Almond Spelt Muffins:** *Add 3/4 cup sliced toasted almonds with the currants. Add 1 teaspoon almond extract with the vanilla.*
>
> **Apricot Pistachio Spelt Muffins:** *Substitute 2/3 cup chopped dried apricots for the currants. Add 1/2 cup shelled unsalted pistachios with the dried apricots.*
>
> **Coconut Spelt Muffins:** *Add 3/4 cup sweetened shredded coconut with the currants.*
>
> **Cranberry Pecan Spelt Muffins:** *Substitute 2/3 cup dried cranberries for the currants. Add 1/2 cup chopped pecans with the cranberries.*
>
> **Date Nut Spelt Muffins:** *Substitute 2/3 cup chopped, pitted dried dates for the currants. Add 1/2 cup chopped walnuts with the dates.*

Sweet Potato Muffins

Makes 12 muffins

Sweet potato pie has long been a Southern favorite, so why not make sweet potato muffins? The roasted sweet potato adds moisture to baked goods and it helps cut down on fat. These are the quintessential muffins, light and beautiful with rounded, cracked tops. Serve them for Thanksgiving breakfast or at brunch any time of the year.

1 large sweet potato (about 1 pound)

Nonstick spray or paper muffin cups

2 cups all-purpose flour

2 teaspoons baking soda

1 teaspoon ground cinnamon

$^1/_2$ teaspoon baking powder

$^1/_2$ teaspoon salt

$^1/_4$ teaspoon grated nutmeg

1 large egg, lightly beaten, at room temperature

6 tablespoons ($^3/_4$ stick) unsalted butter, melted and cooled

$^3/_4$ cup maple syrup, preferably Grade A Dark Amber

$^1/_2$ cup milk (whole or low-fat, but not nonfat)

2 teaspoons lemon juice

1. Position the rack in the center of the oven and preheat the oven to 400°F.

2. Prick the potato in several places with a fork. Lay a piece of aluminum foil on your oven rack to protect your oven from drips, then place the sweet potato on the foil. Bake for 1 hour and 15 minutes, or until soft. Transfer the sweet potato to a wire rack and cool for 10 minutes. Maintain the oven's temperature. (The potato can be baked up to 48 hours ahead of time; cool it completely, tightly wrap it in plastic wrap, and store it in the refrigerator.)

3. Meanwhile, prepare the muffin tins. Spray the indentations and the rims around them with nonstick spray, or line the indentations with paper muffin cups. If using silicon muffin tins, spray as directed, then place the tins on a baking sheet.

4. Whisk the flour, baking soda, cinnamon, baking powder, salt, and nutmeg in a medium bowl until uniform. Set aside.

5. Peel the potato and measure out 1 cup of the cooked flesh; place this amount into a large bowl. (Reserve any additional sweet potato for another use.) Whisk in the egg and melted butter until smooth. Whisk in the maple syrup, milk, and lemon juice. Stir in the flour mixture with a wooden spoon only until moistened, but also so that the batter is uniform with no streaks of sweet potato.

6. Fill the prepared tins three-quarters full. Use additional greased tins or small, oven-safe, greased ramekins for any leftover batter, or reserve the batter for a second baking. Bake for 20 minutes, or until the muffins are well browned, with rounded, cracked tops. A toothpick inserted in the center of one muffin should come out with a few moist crumbs attached.

7. Set the pan on a wire rack to cool for 10 minutes. Gently rock each muffin back and forth to release and remove it from the tin. Cool the muffins for 5 minutes more on the rack before serving. If storing or freezing them, cool them completely before sealing in an airtight container or in freezer-safe plastic bags. The muffins will stay fresh for up to 2 days at room temperature or up to 3 months in the freezer.

Cherry Sweet Potato Muffins: *Add 2/3 cup chopped dried cherries with the flour.*

Honey Sweet Potato Muffins: *Reduce the maple syrup to 1/4 cup. Add 1/2 cup honey with the remaining maple syrup.*

Pecan Sweet Potato Muffins: *Add 2/3 cup chopped pecans with the flour.*

Pumpkin Seed Sweet Potato Muffins: *Add 2/3 cup shelled pumpkin seeds (pepitas) with the flour.*

Sweet Potato Casserole Muffins: *Add 1/2 cup mini marshmallows and 1/3 cup chopped dried pineapple with the flour.*

Sweet Potato Cinnamon Crunch Muffins: *Top the muffins with Cinnamon Sugar Topping (page 225) before baking.*

Sweet Potato Nut Crunch Muffins: *Top the muffins with Nut Crunch Topping (page 229) before baking.*

Vanilla Glazed Sweet Potato Muffins: *Coat the cooled muffins with Vanilla Dip (page 231).*

Tomato Muffins

Makes 12 muffins

The best way to get tomato flavor into a savory muffin is to use canned tomato soup—but that means you should use a quality brand, not one leadened with sweeteners and preservatives. These muffins are orange with the slight tang of cheese, so they are reminiscent of Cheez-It crackers. Give them to your kids as a snack when you want them to cut down on sweets.

Nonstick spray or paper muffin cups
2 cups all-purpose flour
1/4 cup yellow or white cornmeal
1/4 cup sugar
2 teaspoons baking soda
1 teaspoon baking powder
1/2 teaspoon salt
2 large eggs, at room temperature
One 10^3/4-ounce can condensed tomato soup
8 tablespoons (1 stick) unsalted butter, melted and cooled
2 teaspoons lemon juice
1/4 cup grated Parmigiano-Reggiano (1 ounce)

1. Position the rack in the center of the oven and preheat the oven to 400°F. To prepare the muffin tins, spray the indentations and the rims around them with nonstick spray, or line the indentations with paper muffin cups. If using silicon muffin tins, spray as directed, then place them on a baking sheet.

2. Whisk the flour, cornmeal, sugar, baking soda, baking powder, and salt in a medium bowl until well combined. Set aside.

3. In a large bowl, whisk the eggs until lightly beaten, then whisk in the tomato soup, melted butter, and lemon juice. Stir in the cheese, then add the flour mixture, stirring only until moistened but of a uniform color. Do not overmix.

4. Fill the prepared tins three-quarters full. Use additional greased tins or small, oven-safe, greased ramekins for any leftover batter, or reserve the batter for a second bak-

ing. Bake for 18 minutes, or until the muffins have bumpy, rounded tops and a toothpick inserted in the center of one muffin comes out with a few moist crumbs attached.

5. Set the pan on a wire rack to cool for 10 minutes. Gently rock each muffin back and forth to release and remove it from the pan. Cool the muffins for 5 minutes more on the rack before serving. If storing or freezing the muffins, cool completely before sealing in an airtight container or in freezer-safe plastic bags. The muffins will stay fresh for up to 24 hours at room temperature or up to 2 months in the freezer.

> **Cheddar Tomato Muffins:** *Substitute shredded Cheddar for the Parmigiano-Reggiano.*
>
> **Chunky Tomato Muffins:** *Add 1/2 cup marinated sun-dried tomatoes, drained and chopped, with the cheese.*
>
> **Herbed Tomato Muffins:** *Add 2 teaspoons chopped fresh basil, 2 teaspoons chopped fresh oregano, and 1 teaspoon fresh thyme with the salt.*
>
> **Olive Tomato Muffins:** *Add 1/2 cup sliced pitted olives (green or black) with the cheese.*

Walnut Muffins

Makes 12 muffins

Walnut oil is rich in Omega-3 fatty acids, making it a healthy alternative to butter in baking. Along with brown sugar and maple syrup, the oil gives these muffins a golden brown color as well as a flavor that can't be matched. These muffins can be served at lunch or dinner, but they're still at home on the breakfast table alongside a jar of jam.

Nonstick spray or paper muffin cups
1 cup chopped walnut pieces
1^3/4 cups all-purpose flour
2 teaspoons baking powder
^{1}/2 teaspoon salt
2 large eggs, at room temperature
^{1}/4 cup packed light brown sugar
^{1}/2 cup maple syrup
^{1}/2 cup milk (whole, low-fat, or nonfat)
6 tablespoons walnut oil
1 teaspoon vanilla extract

1. Position the rack in the center of the oven and preheat the oven to 400°F.

2. Place the walnut pieces on a baking sheet and bake for 6 minutes, stirring occasionally until lightly brown and fragrant. Transfer the nuts to a large plate and cool for 10 minutes. Maintain the oven's temperature.

3. Meanwhile, prepare the muffin tins. Spray the indentations and the rims around them with nonstick spray, or line the indentations with paper muffin cups. If using silicon muffin tins, spray as directed, then place them on a baking sheet.

4. Pour ^{1}/2 cup of the toasted nuts into a food processor fitted with the chopping blade. Pulse the machine 5 or 6 times until the nuts are finely ground. Do not grind to a paste.

5. Transfer the ground nuts to a medium mixing bowl; add the remaining toasted nuts. Stir in the flour, baking powder, and salt until well combined. Set aside.

6. In a large bowl, whisk the eggs until lightly beaten, then add the brown sugar and maple syrup. Continue whisking until the mixture is thick and pale brown, about 3 minutes. Whisk in the milk, oil, and vanilla until smooth. Using a wooden spoon, stir in the flour mixture until absorbed.

7. Fill the prepared tins three-quarters full. Use additional greased tins or small, oven-safe, greased ramekins for any leftover batter, or reserve the batter for a second baking. Bake for 20 minutes, or until the muffins are golden brown with high, rounded, cracked tops. A toothpick inserted into the center of one muffin should come out clean.

8. Set the pan on a wire rack to cool for 10 minutes. Gently rock each muffin back and forth to release and remove it from the pan. Cool the muffins for 5 minutes more on the rack before serving. If storing or freezing the muffins, cool completely before sealing in an airtight container or in freezer-safe plastic bags. The muffins will stay fresh for up to 2 days at room temperature or up to 3 months in the freezer.

> **Banana Walnut Muffins:** *Add 1/3 cup chopped dried banana with the flour.*
>
> **Cinnamon Crunch Walnut Muffins:** *Top the muffins with Cinnamon Sugar Topping (page 225) before baking.*
>
> **Honey Walnut Muffins:** *Reduce the maple syrup to 1/4 cup. Add 1/4 cup honey with the remaining syrup.*
>
> **Orange Walnut Muffins:** *Reduce the maple syrup to 6 tablespoons. Add 2 tablespoons thawed frozen orange juice concentrate with the remaining syrup.*
>
> **Spiced Cranberry Walnut Muffins:** *Add 1 teaspoon ground cinnamon, 1/4 teaspoon ground mace, and 1/4 teaspoon ground cloves with the flour. Coarsely chop 1/2 cup dried cranberries, then gently press them onto the tops of the muffins before baking.*
>
> **Walnut Crumb Muffins:** *Top the muffins with Crumb Topping (page 226) before baking.*

White Chocolate Muffins

Makes 12 muffins

Wh ite chocolate is simply cocoa butter with no cocoa solids. Unfortunately, some brands, to cut costs, use hydrogenated oil as a filler. For the best taste, read the labels carefully and use a brand of white chocolate that doesn't stretch the mix with additives. While white chocolate is often available in the baking aisle, better brands are sometimes kept in the candy aisle. White chocolate chips will also work.

Nonstick spray or paper muffin cups
2 cups all-purpose flour
1 tablespoon baking powder
$^1/_2$ teaspoon salt
12 ounces white chocolate, finely chopped, or 12 ounces white chocolate chips
4 tablespoons ($^1/_2$ stick) unsalted butter, at room temperature
1 large egg, at room temperature
$^3/_4$ cup sugar
$^3/_4$ cup milk (whole or low-fat, but not nonfat)
1 teaspoon vanilla extract

1. Position the rack in the center of the oven and preheat the oven to 375°F. To pre-pare the muffin tins, spray the indentations and the rims around them with nonstick spray, or line the indentations with paper muffin cups. If using silicon muffin tins, spray as directed, then place them on a baking sheet.

2. Whisk the flour, baking powder, and salt in a medium bowl until uniform. Set aside.

3. Place 4 ounces of the white chocolate and all the butter in the top of a double boiler set over simmering water. If you don't have a double boiler, place the chocolate and butter in a heatsafe bowl that fits snugly over a small pot of simmering water. Stir constantly until half the chocolate and butter is melted. Remove the top of the dou-ble boiler or the bowl from the pot; then continue stirring, away from the heat, until the mixture is smooth. Cool for 10 minutes.

4. In a large bowl, whisk the egg and sugar until thick and pale yellow, about 2 min-utes. Whisk in the cooled chocolate mixture until smooth, then whisk in the milk and vanilla extract.

5. Use a wooden spoon to stir in the remaining chopped white chocolate or white chocolate chips. Stir in the prepared flour mixture just until moistened.

6. Fill the prepared tins three-quarters full. Use additional greased tins or small, oven-safe, greased ramekins for any leftover batter, or reserve the batter for a second baking. Bake for 20 minutes, or until the muffins are browned with slightly rounded tops, and a toothpick inserted in the center of one muffin comes out with a crumb or two attached.

7. Set the pan on a wire rack to cool for 10 minutes. Gently rock each muffin back and forth to release and remove it from the pan. Cool the muffins for 5 minutes more on the rack before serving. If storing or freezing the muffins, cool completely before sealing in an airtight container or in freezer-safe plastic bags. The muffins will stay fresh for up to 24 hours at room temperature or up to 2 months in the freezer.

Black and White Chocolate Muffins: *Top the cooled muffins with Chocolate Icing (page 223).*

White Chocolate Hazelnut Muffins: *Reduce the white chocolate to 8 ounces. Add 2/3 cup chopped toasted hazelnuts with the remaining white chocolate.*

White Chocolate Lemon Muffins: *Add 2 teaspoons lemon extract or 1/2 teaspoon lemon oil with the vanilla. Top the cooled muffins with Lemon Drizzle (page 227).*

White Chocolate Nut Crunch Muffins: *Top the muffins with Nut Crunch Topping (page 229) before baking.*

White Chocolate Oat Crunch Muffins: *Top the muffins with Oat Crunch Topping (page 230) before baking.*

White Chocolate Orange Muffins: *Add 2 teaspoons orange extract or 1/2 teaspoon orange oil with the vanilla.*

White Chocolate Raspberry Muffins: *Reduce the white chocolate to 8 ounces. Gently fold 1/2 cup fresh raspberries into the batter with the prepared flour mixture.*

Whole Wheat Muffins

Makes 12 muffins

If you like simple, relatively healthy muffins, look no further. The large amount of whole wheat flour in this batter produces classic muffins with high, cracked tops, a light tan color, and a soft crumb.

Nonstick spray or paper muffin cups
1³/₄ cups whole wheat flour
³/₄ cup all-purpose flour
1 tablespoon baking powder
¹/₂ teaspoon salt
2 large eggs, at room temperature
¹/₃ cup honey
¹/₃ cup maple syrup
³/₄ cup milk (whole, low-fat, or nonfat)
¹/₃ cup canola oil or vegetable oil
2 teaspoons vanilla extract

1. Position the rack in the center of the oven and preheat the oven to 400°F. To prepare the muffin tins, spray the indentations and the rims around them with nonstick spray, or line the indentations with paper muffin cups. If using silicon muffin tins, spray as directed, then place them on a baking sheet.

2. Whisk the whole wheat flour, all-purpose flour, baking powder, and salt in a medium bowl until well combined. Set aside.

3. In a large bowl, whisk the eggs until lightly beaten, then whisk in the honey and maple syrup until smooth, about 30 seconds. Whisk in the milk, oil, and vanilla. Finally, stir in the prepared flour mixture until incorporated.

4. Fill the prepared tins three-quarters full. Use additional greased tins or small, oven-safe, greased ramekins for any leftover batter, or reserve the batter for a second baking. Bake for 22 minutes, or until the muffins have rounded, cracked tops and a toothpick inserted in the center of one muffin comes out with a few moist crumbs attached.

5. Set the pan on a wire rack to cool for 10 minutes. Gently rock each muffin back and forth to release and remove it from the pan. Cool the muffins for 5 minutes more on the rack before serving. If storing or freezing the muffins, cool completely before sealing in an airtight container or in freezer-safe plastic bags. The muffins will stay fresh for up to 24 hours at room temperature or up to 3 months in the freezer.

> **Chocolate Iced Whole Wheat Muffins:** *Top the cooled muffins with Chocolate Icing (page 223).*
>
> **Oat Crunch Whole Wheat Muffins:** *Top the muffins with Oat Crunch Topping (page 230) before baking.*
>
> **Whole Wheat Butter-Topped Muffins:** *Melt 2 tablespoons unsalted butter. Brush the muffin tops with the melted butter after they've baked for 18 minutes. Continue baking as directed.*
>
> **Whole Wheat Chocolate Chip Muffins:** *Mix 1 cup semisweet chocolate chips into the batter after the flour mixture.*
>
> **Whole Wheat Cinnamon Raisin Muffins:** *Add 1 teaspoon ground cinnamon and 1/2 cup raisins with the whole wheat flour.*
>
> **Whole Wheat Cranberry Walnut Muffins:** *Add 1/3 cup dried cranberries and 1/3 cup chopped walnuts along with the whole wheat flour.*
>
> **Whole Wheat Crumb Muffins:** *Top the muffins with Crumb Topping (page 226) before baking.*
>
> **Whole Wheat Jam Muffins:** *Fill the muffin tins one-third full; gently spread the batter to the rims. Add 1 teaspoon jam to each muffin, then divide the remaining batter equally among the tins, covering the jam.*

Wild Rice Muffins

Makes 12 muffins

Wild rice is not really rice at all—rather, it's the seed of a marsh grass cultivated for centuries by Native Americans in what's now the Upper Midwest. These savory muffins really highlight the nutty taste of wild rice, spiking it with a bit of cheese and a little rye flour. The muffins' crunchy bite makes them a great side dish to a bowl of hot tomato soup or a bowl of cold gazpacho.

$^2/_3$ cup wild rice

2 cups water

Nonstick spray or paper muffin cups

$1^1/_3$ cups all-purpose flour

$^1/_3$ cup rye flour (see Note)

$^1/_3$ cup grated Parmigiano-Reggiano (about $1^1/_2$ ounces)

2 tablespoons sugar

2 teaspoons baking powder

$^1/_2$ teaspoon salt

$^1/_4$ teaspoon grated nutmeg

1 large egg, at room temperature

$^1/_3$ cup milk (whole, low-fat, or nonfat)

$^1/_4$ cup canola or vegetable oil

1. Combine the wild rice and water in a small saucepan; bring the mixture to a boil over high heat. Reduce the heat to very low, cover, and simmer for 45 minutes, or until the wild rice is tender. There will be water remaining; this will be used as liquid in the batter. Let the rice stand away from the heat for 15 minutes, covered.

2. Meanwhile, position the rack in the center of the oven and preheat the oven to 400°F. To prepare the muffin tins, spray the indentations and the rims around them with nonstick spray, or line the indentations with paper muffin cups. If using silicon muffin tins, spray as directed, then place them on a baking sheet.

3. Whisk the all-purpose flour, rye flour, grated cheese, sugar, baking powder, salt, and nutmeg in a medium bowl until well combined. Set aside.

4. In a large bowl, whisk the egg until lightly beaten, then whisk in the milk and oil. Use a wooden spoon to stir in the wild rice and any remaining water in the saucepan until well blended. Stir in the prepared flour mixture until the wild rice is distributed evenly throughout the batter. Do not overmix.

5. Fill the prepared tins to the top with batter. Bake for 16 minutes, or until the muffins have firm tops and a toothpick inserted in the center of one muffin comes out clean.

6. Set the pan on a wire rack to cool for 10 minutes. Gently tip each muffin to one side to make sure it isn't stuck. If one is, rock it back and forth to release it from the pan. Cool the muffins for 5 minutes more on the rack before serving. If storing or freezing the muffins, cool completely before sealing in an airtight container or in freezer-safe plastic bags. The muffins will stay fresh for up to 24 hours at room temperature or up to 2 months in the freezer.

Note: *Since rye flour has far fewer glutens than wheat flour, it is too heavy to make an effective quick bread on its own. However, if added sparingly, it will make a dense, chewy muffin, in keeping with the texture of wild rice. Use only medium or light rye flour, not dark rye or pumpernickel flour.*

Wild Rice Chestnut Muffins: *Add 1 cup roasted, peeled, chopped chestnuts with the cooked wild rice.*

Wild Rice Cranberry Muffins: *Add 3/4 cup dried cranberries with the cooked wild rice.*

Wild Rice Sage Muffins: *Add 2 tablespoons chopped fresh sage with the cooked wild rice.*

Zucchini Muffins

Makes 12 muffins

Zucchini bread is one of those '70s fads that came to stay. Zucchini adds a lot of moisture to a batter, creating hearty, sweet muffins with beautiful flecks of green. Great for backpacking or camping trips, these muffins will stay fresh and moist longer than most.

Nonstick spray or paper muffin cups
$1^2/_3$ cups all-purpose flour
$^1/_2$ cup whole wheat flour
$^1/_3$ cup sugar
1 tablespoon baking powder
$^1/_2$ teaspoon ground ginger
$^1/_2$ teaspoon salt
2 large eggs, at room temperature
$^1/_3$ cup packed light brown sugar
$^1/_4$ cup canola or vegetable oil
$^2/_3$ cup milk (whole, low-fat, or nonfat)
2 teaspoons vanilla extract
2 medium zucchini (about 6 ounces each), washed

1. Position the rack in the center of the oven and preheat the oven to 400°F. To prepare the muffin tins, spray the indentations and the rims around them with nonstick spray, or line the indentations with paper muffin cups. If using silicon muffin tins, spray as directed, then place them on a baking sheet.

2. Whisk the all-purpose flour, whole wheat flour, sugar, baking powder, ground ginger, and salt in a medium bowl until uniform. Set aside.

3. In a large bowl, whisk the eggs until lightly beaten, then add the brown sugar and oil. Continue whisking until the mixture is thick and pale brown, about 2 minutes. Whisk in the milk and vanilla extract.

4. Using the large holes of a box grater, grate the zucchini directly into the wet ingredients; stir until well blended. Then stir in the prepared flour mixture only until

moistened and the zucchini is evenly distributed throughout the batter. Do not overmix.

5. Fill the prepared tins three-quarters full. Use additional greased tins or small, oven-safe, greased ramekins for any leftover batter, or reserve the batter for a second baking. Bake for 25 minutes, or until the muffins have firm rounded tops and a toothpick inserted in the center of one muffin comes out with a few moist crumbs attached.

6. Set the pan on a wire rack to cool for 10 minutes. Gently rock each muffin back and forth to release and remove it from the pan. Cool the muffins for 5 minutes more on the rack before serving. If storing or freezing the muffins, cool completely before sealing in an airtight container or in freezer-safe plastic bags. The muffins will stay fresh for up to 2 days at room temperature or up to 3 months in the freezer.

Zucchini Almond Muffins: *Substitute almond oil for the canola oil. Sprinkle the top of each muffin with 2 teaspoons sliced almonds before baking.*

Zucchini Ginger Walnut Muffins: *Add 1/3 cup chopped walnut pieces and 1/4 cup finely chopped crystallized ginger with the all-purpose flour.*

Zucchini Oat Muffins: *Substitute oat flour for the whole wheat flour. Sprinkle the top of each muffin with 2 teaspoons rolled oats (do not use quick-cooking oats) before baking.*

Zucchini Pecan Muffins: *Add 1/2 cup chopped pecans with the all-purpose flour.*

Zucchini Sunflower Seed Muffins: *Add 1/2 cup shelled sunflower seeds with the all-purpose flour.*

Toppings

The difference between a muffin and a cupcake is also a matter of the toppings. Cupcakes often feature buttercreams or cream cheese frostings. Muffins, however, hold up lighter fare, like an oat crunch or a crumb topping. And while cupcakes are always iced after they're baked, there are two kinds of muffin toppings: baked onto the muffins, or iced on after the muffins have cooled.

In the variations to the muffin recipes, we've listed what we consider the good possibilities for each muffin. But in truth, and within reason, most toppings will work with most muffins. So experiment and see what you can come up with. Our muffins were developed to go it alone, without a topping—but just dress one up and it's guaranteed to make your morning, if not your day.

Chocolate Crunch Topping

Makes a little over 1 cup, enough for 12 muffins

This sweet topping is easy to make; it's a great addition to any chocolate or nut muffin.

$^1/_2$ cup sugar
4 tablespoons ($^1/_2$ stick) unsalted butter, melted and cooled
$^1/_4$ cup cocoa powder, sifted
2 tablespoons all-purpose flour

1. Combine the sugar and butter in small bowl; stir with a fork until blended. Sprinkle the cocoa powder and flour over the top. Stir until the mixture can be pressed into clumps with your fingers.

2. Before baking, sprinkle the topping evenly on the muffin tops by squeezing and crumbling the mixture between your fingers, using approximately 2 tablespoons per muffin.

Chocolate Icing

Makes about 1 1/4 cups, enough for 12 muffins

This fudgy icing makes a luxurious addition to any muffin. It's best applied within an hour of when it's made, although it will keep for up to 1 day at room temperature.

2 ounces unsweetened chocolate, chopped
1/4 cup water
2 tablespoons light corn syrup
1/4 teaspoon salt
2 1/2 cups confectioners' sugar
1/2 teaspoon vanilla extract

1. Place the chocolate in a medium bowl and set aside.

2. Combine the water, corn syrup, and salt in a small saucepan; stir until the salt dissolves. Set the pan over medium heat. Do not stir—the moment the mixture comes to a simmer, remove the pan from the heat. Pour the hot syrup over the chopped chocolate and stir until the chocolate has melted. Cool for 3 minutes, then stir in the confectioner's sugar until a smooth icing begins to form. Add the vanilla and stir until incorporated.

3. Spread about 1 1/2 tablespoons icing on each cooled muffin using a spoon or rubber spatula. Alternatively, dip the cooled muffin tops into the chocolate icing, allowing any excess to drip back into the bowl, then turn the muffin right side up and allow the icing to cool and set before serving.

Cinnamon Streusel Topping

Makes about 3/4 cup, enough for 12 muffins

Streusel is one of the most common muffin toppings. Our version is a flour mixture which cools into a crunchy, sweet, marbleized cinnamon topping. It may insulate the muffins somewhat, requiring a slightly longer baking time, usually about 2 minutes.

1/4 cup all-purpose flour
1/4 cup sugar
1 teaspoon ground cinnamon
4 tablespoons (1/2 stick) unsalted butter, cold

1. Whisk the flour, sugar, and cinnamon in a small bowl until uniform. Slice the butter into 6 equal pieces and add it to the bowl. With a pastry cutter or two forks, cut the butter into the dry ingredients until the mixture resembles coarse meal.

2. Sprinkle the topping evenly on top of the muffins before baking, using approximately 1 tablespoon on each, squeezing and crumbling the mixture between your fingers as you sprinkle.

Cinnamon Sugar Topping

Makes about 1/4 cup, enough for 12 muffins

Cinnamon toast is one of life's pleasures. While this topping is for muffins, not bread, the results are just as euphoric.

1/4 cup sugar
1 1/2 teaspoons ground cinnamon
1 tablespoon unsalted butter, melted and cooled

1. In a small bowl, mix the sugar and cinnamon with a fork until well blended. Add the melted butter and stir until uniform.

2. Before baking, sprinkle evenly on top of your muffins, approximately 1 teaspoon on each.

> **You can vary this topping endlessly by reducing the ground cinnamon to 1 teaspoon and adding 1/2 teaspoon of any of the following:** *ground ginger, grated nutmeg, ground mace, ground cardamom, or ground cloves.*

Crumb Topping

Makes about $^1/_2$ cup, enough for 12 muffins

This basic topping is made with bread crumbs for a light, crunchy, and not-too-sweet cap on any muffin.

2 tablespoons unsalted butter, melted and cooled
2 tablespoons packed light brown sugar
$^1/_4$ cup plain dry breadcrumbs
2 teaspoons all-purpose flour

1. Stir the melted butter and sugar with a fork in a small bowl until blended. Stir in the breadcrumbs and flour until the mixture can be pressed into clumps between your fingers.

2. Before baking, sprinkle the topping evenly on the muffin tops by squeezing and crumbling the mixture between your fingers, using approximately 2 teaspoons per muffin.

Lemon Drizzle

Makes about 1/3 cup, enough for 12 muffins

Acid keeps sugar from crystallizing, so the lemon juice in this recipe keeps the sugar in a semi-liquid form. It's perfect for drizzling designs on the tops of baked muffins.

3/4 cup confectioners' sugar
1 tablespoon lemon juice
1 teaspoon grated lemon zest

1. Stir the confectioners' sugar, lemon juice, and zest in a small bowl until the sugar dissolves and the mixture is smooth. Set aside for 15 minutes to firm up a bit.

2. Drizzle approximately 1 teaspoon on top of each cooled, baked muffin. Alternatively, dip the cooled muffin tops into the drizzle, allow all the excess to drip back off, then turn the muffin right side up and allow the drizzle to set.

Low–Fat Streusel Topping

Makes about ¹/2 cup, enough for 12 muffins

Here's a way to top muffins without blowing your diet.

¹/4 cup packed light brown sugar
3 tablespoons all–purpose flour
¹/2 teaspoon ground cinnamon
1 tablespoon unsalted butter, melted and cooled

1. Combine the brown sugar, flour, and cinnamon in a small bowl. Stir in the melted butter until the mixture can be pressed together into clumps between your fingers.

2. Before baking, sprinkle the topping evenly on the muffin tops by squeezing and crumbling the mixture between your fingers, using approximately 2 teaspoons per muffin.

Nut Crunch Topping

Makes about 1 cup, enough for 12 muffins

As this topping bakes, the nuts toast and the sugar caramelizes. The result is much like nut brittle.

$^1/_2$ cup packed light brown sugar
3 tablespoons unsalted butter, melted and cooled
$^1/_3$ cup finely chopped nuts (such as pecans, walnuts, or almonds)
1 tablespoon plus 1 teaspoon all-purpose flour

1. In a small bowl, stir the sugar and butter with a fork until well combined. Add the nuts and flour; stir until the mixture can be pressed together into clumps between your fingers.

2. Before baking, sprinkle the topping evenly on the muffin tops by squeezing and crumbling the mixture between your fingers, using approximately 1$^1/_2$ tablespoons per muffin.

Oat Crunch Topping

Makes a little over 1 cup, enough for 12 muffins

Here's a topping that's somewhat reminiscent of oatmeal cookies. There's hardly a sweet muffin in this book that wouldn't benefit from it.

$1/4$ cup packed light brown sugar
4 tablespoons ($1/2$ stick) unsalted butter, melted and cooked
6 tablespoons all-purpose flour
$1/4$ cup rolled oats (not quick-cooking oats)
$1/4$ teaspoon grated nutmeg

1. Combine the sugar and butter in a medium bowl; stir with a fork until blended. Stir in the flour, oats, and nutmeg until the mixture can be pressed together into clumps between your fingers.

2. Before baking, sprinkle the topping evenly on the muffin tops by squeezing and crumbling the mixture between your fingers, using approximately 2 teaspoons per muffin.

Vanilla Dip

Makes about 1/2 cup, enough for 12 muffins

This is a simple icing for baked muffins. Don't spread it with a knife—just dip the baked and cooled muffin tops into this thin glaze until they're lightly coated, as if you were gently dipping something into thin paint. The topping will be soft when set.

2 tablespoons water
2 teaspoons light corn syrup
1/8 teaspoon salt
1 teaspoon vanilla extract
1 1/4 cups confectioners' sugar

1. Stir the water, corn syrup, and salt in a small saucepan until the salt dissolves. Place the pan over medium heat and bring to a simmer without stirring. Once it simmers, remove at once from the heat and stir in the vanilla extract. Stir in the sugar in 1/4 cup increments until the dip is smooth. Transfer to a medium bowl to cool slightly, about 5 minutes.

2. Dip the tops of cooled baked muffins into the mixture and let the excess drip back into the bowl. If desired, and if any topping remains, dip the muffins a second time for a thicker glaze. Set the muffins right side up on a plate and allow the dip to set at room temperature for about 15 minutes.

A List of Specialty Muffins

Looking for something special or a way to use a special ingredient you have on hand? These lists will get you started. Just look under the category that best delivers what you need. We have not included every variation from every muffin, just base recipes and a few variations that you might otherwise miss.

CHOCOLATE AND CHOCOLATE CHIP MUFFINS

Almond Joy Muffins (variation of Almond Muffins), Berries and Chips Muffins (variation of Berry Muffins), Black Forest Muffins, Butterscotch Chocolate Muffins (variation of Butterscotch Muffins), Cherry Chocolate Chip Muffins (variation of Cherry Muffins), Chocolate Angel Food Muffins, Chocolate Chip Cappuccino Muffins (variation of Cappuccino Muffins), Chocolate Chip Coffeecake Muffins (variation of Coffeecake Muffins), Chocolate Chip Graham Cracker Muffins (variation of Graham Cracker Muffins), Chocolate Chip Muffins, Chocolate Chip Sour Cream Muffins (variation of Sour Cream Muffins), Chocolate Chocolate Chip Muffins, Chocolate Coconut Muffins (variation of Coconut Muffins), Chocolate Malt Muffins, Chocolate Chip Marmalade Muffins (variation of Marmalade Muffins), Chocolate Chip Orange Muffins (variation of Orange

Muffins), Chocolate Rice Pudding Muffins (variation of Rice Pudding Muffins), Cocoa Muffins, Cola Muffins, Fudge Muffins, Hazelnut Chocolate Chip Muffins (variation of Hazelnut Muffins), Low-Fat Chocolate Chip Muffins, Mexican Chocolate Chip Margarita Muffins (variation of Margarita Muffins), Mexican Chocolate Muffins, Peanut Butter Chocolate Chip Muffins (variation of Peanut Butter Muffins), Rainbow Muffins (variation of Basic Muffins), Red Velvet Muffins, Rice Flour Chocolate Chip Muffins (variation of Rice Flour Muffins), S'mores Muffins, White Chocolate Cheesecake Muffins (variation of Cheesecake Muffins), and White Chocolate Chip Strawberry Muffins (variation of Strawberry Muffins), and White Chocolate Muffins.

CORNMEAL MUFFINS

Cheddar Muffins, Corn Muffins, Cranberry Muffins, Jalapeño Corn Muffins, Lemon Poppy Seed Muffins, Low-Fat Corn Muffins, Low-Fat Peach Muffins, Margarita Muffins, Nonfat Berry Muffins, Nonfat Corn Muffins, Olive Oil Muffins, Parmesan Cornmeal Muffins (variation of Parmesan Muffins), Peach Muffins, Quiche Lorraine Muffins, and Tomato Muffins.

DAIRY-FREE MUFFINS

Angel Food Muffins, Chocolate Angel Food Muffins, Low-Fat Banana Mango Muffins (variation of Low-Fat Banana Muffins), Low-Fat Triple Banana Muffins (variation of Low-Fat Banana Muffins), Nonfat Corn Muffins, and Sugar-Free Spelt Muffins.

GLUTEN-FREE MUFFINS

Gluten-Free Berry Muffins and Rice Flour Muffins.

LOW-FAT MUFFINS

Applesauce Bran Muffins (variation of Bran Muffins), Chocolate Angel Food Muffins, Heart-Healthy Applesauce Muffins (variation of Applesauce Muffins), Heart-Healthy Muffins (variation of Basic Muffins), Low-Fat Banana Muffins, Low-Fat Berry Muffins, Low-Fat Cherry Muffins, Low-Fat Chocolate Chip Muffins, Low-Fat Corn Muffins,

Low-Fat Peach Muffins, Lychee Muffins (if using nonfat yogurt), Prune Muffins (if using low-fat buttermilk), Reduced-Fat Lemon Poppy Seed Muffins (variation of Lemon Poppy Seed Muffins), Sour Cream Muffins (if using nonfat sour cream and nonfat milk), Sugar-Free Spelt Muffins, and Strawberry Muffins (if using low-fat or nonfat yogurt).

MUFFINS WITH CHEESE

Apple Cheddar Muffins (variation of Apple Muffins), Beer Muffins, Cheddar Muffins, Cheesecake Muffins, Cream Cheese Muffins, Herbed Goat Cheese Olive Oil Muffins (variation of Olive Oil Muffins), Parmesan Muffins, Pear Parmesan Muffins (variation of Pear Muffins), Pine Nut Muffins, Pizza Muffins, Potato Cheese Muffins (variation of Potato Muffins), Quiche Lorraine Muffins, Roasted Garlic Muffins, Stilton Muffins, Tomato Muffins, and Wild Rice Muffins.

MUFFINS WITH HONEY

Almond Muffins, Bran Muffins, Chestnut Honey Muffins (variation of Chestnut Muffins), Date and Honey Matzo Brei Muffins (variation of Matzo Brei Muffins), Earl Grey Tea Muffins, Fig Muffins, Graham Cracker Muffins, Honey Fruitcake Muffins (variation of Fruitcake Muffins), Honey Muffins, Honey Sweet Potato Muffins (variation of Sweet Potato Muffins), Honey Walnut Muffins (variation of Walnut Muffins), Low-Fat Corn Muffins, Refrigerator Honey Bran Muffins, and Whole Wheat Muffins.

NONFAT MUFFINS

Angel Food Muffins, Nonfat Berry Muffins, and Nonfat Corn Muffins.

OAT AND OAT BRAN MUFFINS

Berry Muffins, Earl Grey Tea Muffins, Low-Fat Banana Muffins, Low-Fat Berry Muffins, Nutty Oat Honey Muffins (variation of Honey Muffins), Oat Bran Muffins, Oatmeal Muffins, Pecan Oat Muffins (variation of Pecan Muffins), Refrigerator Oat Bran Muffins, Spelt Muffins, Strawberry Jam Muffins, and Zucchini Oat Muffins (variation of Zucchini Muffins).

SAVORY MUFFINS

Beer Muffins, Cheddar Muffins, Corn Muffins, Jalapeño Corn Muffins, Parmesan Muffins, Pizza Muffins, Potato Muffins, Quiche Lorraine Muffins, Roasted Garlic Muffins, Rye Muffins, Stilton Muffins, Tomato Muffins, and Wild Rice Muffins.

WHOLE WHEAT AND WHEAT BRAN MUFFINS

Bran Muffins, Cherry Muffins, Chestnut Muffins, Date Muffins, Fig Muffins, Hazelnut Muffins, Honey Muffins, Low-Fat Cherry Muffins, Marmalade Muffins, Prune Muffins, Refrigerator Honey Bran Muffins, Refrigerator Oat Bran Muffins, Roasted Garlic Muffins, Whole Wheat Lemon Poppy Seed Muffins (variation of Poppy Seed Muffins), Whole Wheat Muffins, and Zucchini Muffins.

WHEAT-FREE MUFFINS

Gluten-Free Berry Muffins, Rice Flour Muffins, and Sugar-Free Spelt Muffins.

Source Guide

Broadway Panhandler
www.broadwaypanhandler.com
866-COOKWARE or 212-966-3434
477 Broome Street
New York, NY 10013
Muffin tins, mixers, spatulas, wooden spoons, mixing bowls, sifters, and just about anything else you need for making muffins.

Kalustyan's
www.kalustyans.com
212-685-3451
123 Lexington Avenue
New York, NY 10016
The place for international one-stop-shopping, including nut oils, exotic flours, flavorings, and dried fruits.

King Arthur Flour
www.kingarthurflour.com
800-827-6836
Norwich, Vermont
Not only great flour, but a catalog with hard-to-find items like rye flour, cherry or cinnamon chips, and different sizes of paper muffin cups.

Marshall's Honey Farm at the Flying Bee Ranch
www.MarhallsHoney.com
800-624-4637
159 Lombard Road
American Canyon, CA 94503
Great honey of all varieties from family-owned apiaries in northern California.

New York Cake and Baking Distributors
800-942-2539 or 212-675-CAKE
56 West 22nd Street
New York, NY 10010
Every baking tool imaginable.

Penzeys Spices
www.penzeys.com
800-741-7787
19300 Janacek Court
Brookfield, WI 53045
Incredibly fresh spices and some of the best vanilla extract available.

Sur La Table
www.surlatable.com
800-243-0852
Outlets across the country, including
84 Pine Street
Seattle, Washington 98101
Kitchenware and baking supplies for every kitchen.

Williams-Sonoma
www.williams-sonoma.com
800-541-2233
P.O. Box 7456
San Francisco, CA 94120
Mixers, bowls, baking pans, and many flavorings from this national retail chain.

www.ultimatecook.com
Recipes and information on the Ultimate Books, on Bruce and Mark, and a list of links to some of our favorite mail-order sources.

Index

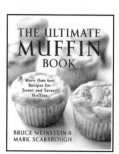
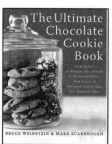
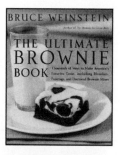
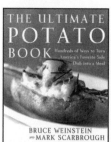
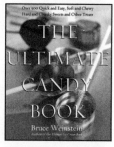
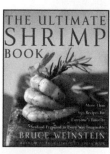
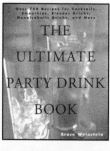
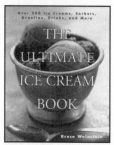